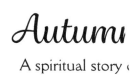

Autumn

A spiritual story

Jim Loch

WEE
JIMMY L
BOOKS

Published in 2016 by Wee Jimmy L Books

ISBN Paperback: 978-0-9954988-0-8
eBook: 978-0-9954988-1-5

A CIP catalogue copy of this book can be
found in the British Library.

Published with the help of Indie Authors World

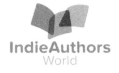

IndieAuthors
World

Dedication

I dedicate this book to Linda, my beautiful soulmate for forty-one years. She enriched my life and the lives of so many people. Her courage and gentle spirit were an inspiration to us all.

I will Remember,
Lift up my heart
and give Thanks.

Acknowledgements

*A*t first, when I considered how to structure this, I looked upon it as a bit of a chore. At the back of my mind was the thought that I didn't want to offend anybody. Consequently, I drew something up that was pretty safe and submitted it. On reflection I found it to be lifeless and I realised that it was not worthy of the book. This is my second attempt and have I decided to follow the spirit of the book, open my heart, address you directly and pour my gratitude out. It is not meant to be all inclusive, so sorry if I have missed mentioning you.

I am so proud of you my family. You were a tower of strength throughout, even although you were scattered throughout the world. Despite Stuart and Jessica living in USA, Fraser and Larinda in Canada and Iain in Australia, we felt your support from the start. It was just wonderful Iain that you were able to come back home to stay with us throughout. It meant so much to us, Stuart and Fraser, for you to bring your families home to visit us during Linda's treatment. Dave, my big brother, you have huge heart and have always been my protector and there you were again in the background, ably supported by your wonderful wife Alison. I love both of you so much. Malcolm and Margaret, thanks for opening your hearts, I felt our relationship grew closer with our shared vulnerability.

Thank you to my wonderful neighbours. Rhona you were just great with your mixture of love, wisdom and practical suggestions. Helen, we really appreciated those wonderful letters of encouragement and William, thanks for being my buddy!

High Blantyre Baptist church folks, you are a tremendously caring little community and we felt you walked with us each step of the way, with love and prayerful support. Special thanks to Steve, Chris, sweet Rebeca, Phil and Janet, the bonds that we have together were fashioned in heaven. Also Steve, thanks for being my rock and leading the funeral services so sensitively. St. Mary's Episcopal church folks, thanks for your love and support too. Iain, your wisdom was much appreciated and Jean, thanks for being my constant companion beside me in the pew.

Linda's work colleagues at Calderside Academy, especially the office staff - thanks for everything, you supported us on our journey and helped make the funeral service special.

Voice Coach Deirdre Trundle (who sadly died in 2013), you have enriched my life in so many ways throughout the years and I owe you a great debt for coaching me through my delivery of Linda's Eulogy. Thanks Doris Simpson for using your considerable talent in playing the piano at the funeral service and accompanying me with my love song.

The medical treatment that Linda received from the NHS was exemplary. I thank you all; the staff at Calderside Health Centre; Mr Murphy the surgeon and his breast cancer team of nurses at Monklands Hospital Airdrie, especially Jackie; Dr Hicks the oncologist and all the staff at the chemotherapy treatment centre at Wishaw General Hospital. A special thanks to all you volunteers and staff at The Haven, especially Marion for using your skills as a hairdresser to help Linda deal with her hair loss.

I would also like to thank - my Counselling Professional Development Group for your encouragement and care for me. Daniel Kish for all your loving support in suggesting alternatives to conventional treatment and Lachlan McIntyre for your invaluable help in my time of need, at the end of Linda's life.

There have also been wonderful souls, who have encouraged me in writing this manuscript and getting it ready for publication.

Thanks to you Fraser and Larinda for coming up with the idea of sending me away on a writer's course for my birthday in Inverness. I found it extremely helpful and met Rosey Bensley, who has become a very close friend and confidant. Both of us had stories to tell, so thanks Rosey for reading and editing my script and allowing me to read and edit yours.

However, the main reason that I have managed to get this book published is because of the personal and professional help of Kim and Sinclair Macleod of Indie Authors World. I cannot thank you enough and it is a joy to have both of you in my life. Special thanks also to Alister Blyth for your sensitivity and professional services in editing my document.

If I have missed you out, please accept my apologies and sincere thanks.

Introduction

I started writing this about one year after Linda died. Five years later it was almost ready to be published, but something about it did not sit well with me. I had been motivated to write it, because so many wonderful things had happened during Linda's illness, eventual death and burial and I wanted to share them with our friends and family.

I had written 20 chapters of our journey together. It would tell *Our Story!* However it gradually dawned on me that it was not *Our Story* at all, but *My Story*. Linda hadn't written any of it; hadn't been consulted and hadn't shared how she felt. It was **my** story of accompanying her throughout this terrible, yet somehow beautiful time.

I have written what I remember and have tried to be honest and accurate. However my memory is fallible and I recognise that others may remember the events differently and that is *Their Story*.

I needed a title and I had been mulling it over in my mind for a few days, when I happened to mention it to Larinda, my daughter in law.

"How about Autumn Leaves?", she suggested with a tear in her eye.

Perfect, I thought.

When I see the autumn leaves, I think of you my Love. Leaves bursting forth into a kaleidoscope of shades of green, red, yellow, orange, brown and purple. Oh how we loved to journey in the autumn of each year to Pitlochry and walk hand in hand along the Pass of Killiecrankie, transfixed by the beauty around us. Autumn sees me return year after year to walk alone, Holly my only companion now. I still feel an acute sense of sadness at your passing, but I am also thankful for having shared so many wonderful years with you.

When I see the autumn leaves it reminds me also that it was in the autumn that you left me, my precious one. Wonderfully, over the years, I have learned to let you go. I want the best for you my beloved, so I let you return to our loving God with my blessing. I journey on now in God's hands, surrounded by my wonderful family and friends and of course, my four footed companion.

I dedicate this piece of writing to you my Love, wherever you are!

Chapter 1
The Journey Begins

*I*t all began in the autumn of 2008. Linda had been complaining of a sore upper arm for a couple of months. She attributed it to the constant stretching to push a button at the reception area of her school office, allowing people access to the building. She consulted a GP at the local health centre and he treated it as a muscle strain.

However when it did not improve Linda made an appointment with Dr Dunn, the head of the practice, on Monday, January 26th 2009. After careful examination, Dr Dunn found a small lump on Linda's lymph nodes under her arm. Somewhat concerned she made an **urgent** referral to the breast clinic at Hairmyers Hospital. I had considerable misgivings about this lump and when no appointment came within a week, I contacted the clinic only to be told that they had not even received the request. I immediately phoned Dr Dunn and she faxed through another urgent request. Meantime Linda made a further appointment to see Dr Dunn on the following Friday. My concern was growing so I resolved to attend with Linda. On the Thursday of that week the breast clinic appointment arrived by post for a date **three weeks later!**

This meant that Linda's waiting time to see a specialist was **five weeks!**

On asking the clinic about the unsatisfactory delay I was shocked to be told that it was because the consultant was on holiday for two weeks – apparently there was **no clinic** when he was away! When we told Dr Dunn on the Friday morning, she too was shocked and promised to complain. Fortunately my background was in the NHS, where I had worked in the medical laboratories for 33 years rising to the post of Chief Technician. I was aware of how the system worked (or didn't in this case) and had a reputation for being able to work with people to resolve situations with minimum fuss. Using the skills I had acquired, I took the matter in hand when we arrived home.

I phoned the clinic and asked if there was any way to expedite the appointment.

A very helpful lady suggested I contact Lanarkshire's other general hospitals (Wishaw and Monklands), to ask if either could see Linda sooner. After drawing a blank with Wishaw, I explained the situation to another helpful lady at Monklands. I was seriously considering arranging a private consultation when she called back to offer Linda an appointment **two days later** on Monday, February 9th at Monklands Hospital.

The delay had been cut from five weeks to two!

We were so thankful and we had the feeling that God was going before us, preparing the way.

The next week was a whirlwind!

Linda was seen at the clinic by a registrar, who immediately referred her to Mr Murphy, the surgeon. He was a very self assured, gracious person and we warmed to him. Although the lump was quite small and possibly not serious, he felt it should be investigated urgently and an ultrasound was arranged for the next day.

The results of that ultrasound were "suspicious", so a mammogram and biopsy were arranged for Thursday and a further appointment was squeezed in to see Mr Murphy on Friday, the day before he went on holiday for a fortnight.

We were now really apprehensive and the diagnosis confirmed our worst fears.

Linda had breast cancer and it had spread to her lymph nodes!

We both knew it was a possibility, but to hear the actual words put us into a state of shock. However Mr Murphy assured us that it was treatable and he sent the biopsy to another laboratory for further analysis. This would help with the choice of chemotherapy, in particular whether hormone treatment was likely to be effective. In the following two weeks Mr Murphy arranged bone and CT scans and gave us an appointment to see him after he returned from holiday on February 23rd. We also met Mary, one of the breast cancer nurses, who gave us information on cancer and the support available.

We were dazed by the rapid turn of events and felt that we had entered another world. We cried much together and resolved that we would face this as a team and overcome it with God's help. Our family and friends were shocked by the news. The question on most of their lips was, "How could this happen to a lovely person like Linda?"

However events also seemed to show God's provision for us. Linda had been very apprehensive about attending the radiography department for the mammogram and biopsy procedures. She had found her previous routine mammogram to be very painful. However this time she was attended by a lovely girl who treated her very gently and professionally, resulting in a pain free procedure. In passing, Linda happened to mention her concerns about the afternoon biopsy. Even although she was off in the afternoon, this wonderful girl offered to stay and hold Linda's hand throughout. Linda accepted her kind offer and it made all the difference. I observed that Linda brought out the best in people. We began to look upon them as *"angels"* sent from above to help us on our way.

We were full of trepidation when we next saw Mr Murphy on February 23rd. The laboratory test results disappointingly showed that hormone treatment was unlikely to work. However he assured us that there were many more agents that could be used and more importantly, the cancer was still treatable. The bone and CT scan results were thankfully negative. There was an unexplained elevated calcium level. The treatment plan was chemotherapy, a mastectomy and finally radiotherapy. Dr Murphy hoped Linda would be "clear by Christmas".

We felt encouraged and an appointment was made to see oncologist Dr Hicks the following day at Wishaw General Hospital. Linda was informed that she would lose her hair and details were given to us of hairdressers who supplied wigs under the NHS.

Dr Hicks turned out to be lovely man who reminded me of Dr Who, a cross between the Tom Baker and David Tennant regenerations. Someone who didn't look like a professional until he started speaking. He explained the timescale of the treatment plan. Linda would have her first chemotherapy session the following week, on March 3rd, the day after her 58th birthday. There would be six sessions and each would be three weeks apart. After a short break to allow her immune system to recover, she would have a total mastectomy and after another short break, the final radiotherapy treatment. He was obviously very competent and experienced and we felt encouraged.

Meantime our support base was being activated.

Our close and extended families rallied round. Iain, our nomadic 27-year-old youngest son arrived from Australia on March 2nd (one day before Linda's chemotherapy started) and promised to stay until the cancer was successfully treated. Our other two sons and their families, Stuart in the USA and Fraser in Canada, pledged their support but understandably it had to be from "afar" in the short term.

High Blantyre Baptist (Linda's church) and Hamilton Episcopal Church (my church) rallied round. Neighbours, Linda's work colleagues, close friends and acquaintances suddenly all became visible to support us.

Linda's prayer partner in the Baptist church was the pastor's son, a lovely young man called Philip. We had known him since he was born and he gave Linda a verse that was to become be a constant source of inspiration to us throughout our journey.

"I say this, because I know what I am planning for you" says the Lord. "I have good plans for you, not plans to hurt you. I will give you hope and a good future." **Jeremiah 29:11**

Linda had never been keen on needles and would feel faint at the sight of blood. However she was surprised at how she was able to tolerate the regular blood samples that were now being taken. Looking back, this was an example of the *"Grace of God"*, given to help negotiate her passage.

Around this time I had contact with a very dear, blind friend of ours, Daniel Kish. He was president of the charity, World Access for the Blind and travelled the world conducting workshops. Daniel was a proponent of the natural health philosophy that advocated the benefits of the consumption of raw food. His blindness had been caused by cancer and he believed that this diet had stopped any spread or recurrence of the disease. He told us there was an alternative to the conventional treatment. It was advocated by the Hippocrates Institute in USA. He put us in touch with a member of his board, Dr Ram Aditya, who offered to coach Linda through the treatment. We had never heard of the diet and considered it briefly, mainly because of our regard for Daniel. However it was foreign to us and given the *"life and death"* issues we were facing, we considered it too risky. We thanked him for his offer of help and explained that we had full confidence in the conventional medical treatment and the team delivering it.

It is also worth stating that at the latter part of my career in the NHS, I had difficulty with anxiety and depression. I tried antidepressants, counselling, relaxation, meditation, massage, cognitive behavioural therapy, and other things, but none had any lasting benefit. This affected me to the point where I resigned from the NHS and was awarded an ill health pension in 1997. However, I had developed a great deal of insight into working with emotions,so I retrained as a counsellor and worked as a volunteer, for five years in the Tom Allan Counselling Centre in Glasgow, and two years part-time, in GP practices in Lanarkshire. I left when my father's health deteriorated and had the privilege of being his carer for the last two years of his life. These experiences were to stand me in good stead as I sought to support Linda.

Chapter 2
March/April '09 - Chemotherapy Begins

*L*inda's treatment regime involved three chemotherapy agents being given one after the other. She had just about finished the first when she felt a tingling sensation. This quickly spread and a nurse recognised it as a very rare allergic reaction. The treatment was stopped. I was shocked to see the reaction make Linda's face age 20 years before my eyes; she became, for a short time, an old woman with wrinkles all over her face! Thankfully after antihistamine treatment, her face returned to normal. No further chemotherapy was given that day and the next session was arranged for three weeks time, when a new regime would be administered.

The chemotherapy unit staff were very kind and supportive and we were thankful to be surrounded by so much love. We looked upon this as a brief setback as we continued on our journey. Linda was measured for a wig later that week. We also heard about The Haven, our local cancer support centre, which happened to be attached to our GP practice and we both enrolled for its services. Linda made an appointment the following Monday to see Marion, a hairdresser at the centre who advised clients about all aspects of hair loss. She turned out to be a very warm, loving person and was one several unpaid Haven volunteers. Linda signed up for aromatherapy sessions and I opted for reflexology. Once again we were so thankful for all God's provision for us.

We tried to maintain as normal a life as possible during this time and on March 19th, after Linda's morning reflexology appointment we visited Callander, one of our favourite places. We had a lovely time, belatedly celebrating Linda's birthday.

On Saturday, March 21st Linda's church held their regular coffee morning. It was quite an emotional experience as many there had not seen Linda since the cancer diagnosis. After the initial emotional contact everyone, including Linda, just rolled up their sleeves and got on with serving as usual. It was lovely and once again we were thankful to have so many wonderful people in our lives.

The next chemotherapy session was scheduled for Tuesday, March 24th and it was with some trepidation that we attended. Thankfully everything went really well and we rejoiced that Linda had started the chemo. She had another five sessions ahead because they would not count the first. The routine at the chemotherapy unit was that firstly Linda would check into outpatient reception and get her blood samples taken. This was done by very experienced nurses, who were highly skilled in the art of phlebotomy. An oncologist would interview us, review treatment and order the chemotherapy agents to be used that day. We would then go to the chemotherapy suite, where we would be given a pager. An hour or two later, when summoned, we would return for Linda to have the treatment. This process would finish around 3pm when we would return home. I had the privilege of being by her side almost all of the time.

The suppression of Linda's bone marrow was a side effect of the chemotherapy. To counteract this she needed the intradermal administration of a substance to stimulate her bone marrow. This was to be done at home daily for seven days after the treatment and the district nurses were informed. They were lovely people and even suggested that I could give her the injections if I wanted to. That way we would not be inconvenienced by having to wait at home for the nurses every day for a week. I was a bit reticent at first, but then opened myself up to the possibility of doing it. Each day I aseptically prepared the injection and gave it to the nurses to administer. To be honest, I could not see myself actually injecting Linda, in case I messed it up and hurt her. On the fourth day, after I prepared the injection, the district nurse turned to me with a twinkle in her eye and said, "Right Jim, you are doing it today!"

I felt extremely nervous, but I swallowed hard and did it! I was so proud of myself and we rejoiced together. In retrospect it turned out to be a precious time for both of us, a time of real intimacy, as I honed my technique to make it as pain free as possible.

As my 60th birthday approached, Linda asked me what I wanted for a gift. I said that I had no idea but would think about it. About a year and a half previously, I had begun what I termed my *musical adventure*. (This is a beautiful story and is told elsewhere). I had found my voice and could now sing as a soloist. Linda had encouraged me by giving me voice coach lessons as a Christmas present. As I was walking my dog Holly first thing in the morning, it came to me what I wanted, as a gift for my birthday. I wanted to sing for my friends. In particular my friends in Linda's church at their anniversary service the day after my birthday.

I also wanted to sing for my friends in my own church at the morning service on the following day.

God had prepared the way for us and a very dear 75-year-old friend, Roger, agreed to help me pick a song and accompany me on the electric piano in Linda's church. We selected a beautiful song by American gospel artist Jessy Dixon, called *'The night before Easter'*.

I enrolled the help of my voice coach and between us we managed to prepare me for this special gift. Linda was lovely through all of this, giving her support at all times. I felt that this turned out to be a useful distraction for us, a bit of normality with a tinge of excitement. Linda's church (which previously had also been my church) still held a special place in my heart and was a small caring community.

The anniversary service was a beautiful experience. It was like a birthday party for me and the church. It was great to be surrounded by so many wonderful caring friends as I shared the lovely song with them. Linda was a little nervous; she felt that I had a good voice but questioned whether I had a soloist's voice. Roger accompanied me beautifully on the piano and we all had a really precious time. The next day I sang the song again, unaccompanied, in my own church in Hamilton. It also went very well and the congregation were very appreciative. We felt blessed to be encompassed by so much love from both fellowships.

Chapter 3
May/June '10 - Chemotherapy Continues

By the end of May Linda was halfway through her chemotherapy. By and large she seemed to tolerate it pretty well. The night after her treatment, she would have trouble sleeping because of the effect of the steroids. Her night would be spent in the reclining chair in our lounge, listening to music on her recently acquired iPod. She also had pains in her legs, for which she took pain killers. Her beautiful hair had gradually fallen out and it was sad for us both to see clumps of it in the shower. However, by this time she had her wig, which she wore in public and a series of scarves to wear in the house. She was just beautiful with and without her hair, as her graciousness and courage shone through. Thankfully, apart from an occasional bout of squeamishness, she had no sickness. The anti-sickness tablets were proving effective.

We met the surgeon on May 18th and he was very pleased with Linda's progress. The lump under her arm had shrunk a bit and everyone was optimistic about the future. The plan was to finish the chemotherapy in July and then allow a few weeks for Linda's system to recover. The total mastectomy would take place in August, followed by six weeks radiotherapy starting in October. We were on target for being "free from cancer by Christmas".

We also got the good news that our middle son Fraser and his family, who had emigrated to Canada, were coming to stay with us for most of June. While we were delighted for them to come, I was worried about the upheaval in the house and the effect it would have on Linda. She was always really tired the first week after chemotherapy. Her fourth round was planned for June 2nd and they were due to arrive on the 7th and leave on the 26th. I shared my concerns with our neighbour Rhona, a constant source of encouragement, support and wisdom in our journey. She came up with a wonderful solution. Her next door neighbours, Robert and Christine at No 27, always spent the whole of June in their residential caravan in St Annes, near Blackpool. Perhaps they would let us use their house when they were away. Rhona spoke to them on our behalf and they gladly put their home at our disposal. The plan was that Linda and I would sleep there and Iain, Fraser and his family would all stay in our house. What a weight came off my shoulders and we thanked God for giving us such considerate neighbours.

Linda's fourth round of chemotherapy went according to plan and she coped pretty well with the side effects. She did as best as she could to rest, so that she would be at her best when the visitors arrived. However Linda liked to be organised and so it was a real team effort with Linda directing, and Iain and I being the labourers. Iain was wonderful through all of this; solid and dependable with a big open heart. This wee, cheeky faced, mischievous individual, who as a baby we had bathed in the kitchen sink, had turned into a wonderful young man.

Fraser, Larinda and their children, Nathanael, Ethan and Hannah, all duly arrived at Glasgow Airport. Iain and I drove them to our home. It was a very emotional reunion for us all. Four years previously, it tore our hearts out when they emigrated. We had visited them twice in Canada, but we had never seen Hannah, as she was only seven months old. We had a lovely time together and the accommodation plans worked a treat.

Linda and I would spend the late mornings, afternoons and evenings with our visitors. Around 10pm we would retire to

No 27, have a leisurely supper and talk over the happenings of our day. We would usually be pretty tired so we slept well. In the morning we would rise and have a peaceful breakfast in the lovely conservatory, before returning refreshed to our own house. If at any time Linda felt too tired during the day, she would just go to No 27 and rest.

It was great to do normal things in our house together and treasure each other as we were doing them. We had lots of "wee runs" to our favourite local beauty spots, Callander, Bothwell Castle, Dollar Glen, Chatelherault Country Park, to name a few. We found we had a new attitude to time now and lived more in the present. Linda loved having her grandchildren around her and they were having the time of their lives with "Granny Linda". She had such a big heart of unconditional love and it was a joy to see them interacting. Hannah was a wee stunner; a right wee cutie. For three generations in the Loch household there were only sons and it was a joy to have a wee girl at last for Linda to nurture.

Alas, time sped by and it was time to part. Linda wisely decided to say her farewells at home. Many tears were shed on parting. It reminded me of the time four years before when they emigrated. We consoled ourselves with promises to visit them next year in Canada, once Linda's cancer had been treated successfully. Iain and I drove them to the airport and more tears rolled.

It was around this time that Daniel Kish came back into our lives. I had for some time been having trouble with urinary frequency. I had been diagnosed as having an overactive bladder with an enlarged prostate. No medication had any appreciable benefit. I also tried one or two alternative therapies with the same outcome. A referral to an endocrinologist had revealed no abnormalities. I was left just to manage it myself and I was becoming a bit disenchanted with the medical profession. It was proving troublesome at times, especially when I had to leave Linda's side to find the nearest toilet.

Daniel had maintained an interest in Linda's progress and I asked if his raw food diet might benefit me. I was put back in contact with Ram who assured me that the raw food diet would help. He was so confident that he offered a contract whereby if there was no benefit there would be no charge. I discussed it with Linda and we agreed that I should allow Ram to coach me.

I had a secondary reason for trying it. It would give us some experience of the raw food diet should the conventional treatment be ineffective. Coaching with Ram began with a colonic cleansing programme and teaching sessions before going on the diet. My urination frequency problem worsened. Ram assured us that these symptoms were only temporary and so I persevered and started the diet.

When I began the programme I weighed 9 stone 10 lbs. After three weeks on the programme and only three days on the actual diet, I was 9 stone 2 lbs. Linda freaked out, demanding I come off the diet. After discussing it with Ram I decided to terminate the programme. Linda assured me that after she was "better", if I still wanted to, she would support me in the raw food diet. I felt really bad about placing excess strain on Linda at this very vulnerable time for her. However she did not hold it against me and we recommitted ourselves, as a team, to our fight against the cancer.

On June 30th Linda's fifth chemotherapy session passed without incident. There was only one more session left.

Throughout this time we had a continued awareness that we were building special relationships with so many people. Our neighbours, who we had known for years, supported us tremendously. Nothing was too much trouble. We opened our hearts to each other and a new closeness developed. Helen, across in No 26, had a special gift for writing letters of encouragement and from time to time one slipped through our letterbox. We read them and once again thanked God for motivating her in this way.

Chapter 4
July/August – Chemotherapy ends / Mastectomy

On July 21st Linda had her sixth and final chemotherapy session. It seemed to go smoothly and we rejoiced together. The first lap of the journey had been successfully negotiated!

On August 3rd we had a routine appointment with Mr Murphy. Linda's arm, the one with the affected lymph nodes, was a bit swollen and we wondered why. He put it down to excess fluid being produced but did not seem too worried about it and referred Linda to a clinic to be measured for a special sleeve, which would help to bring the swelling down. As an alternative, he suggested that a specialist in lymphatic massage might be worth consulting.

We tried one or two contacts to find a masseur but drew a blank. However as regards the special sleeve, God seemed to go before us, preparing the way. It was a really busy clinic with a long waiting list, but after a telephone call, they managed to squeeze Linda in later on that week. The technician who attended Linda ended up doing it on her lunch hour. She was another lovely person, taking the measurements and ordering the sleeve. It would be ready the following week and as she had no appointments free, she willingly consented to do it in her lunch hour again. I remember her twinkling eye and conspiratorial voice, "Don't tell the clerical officer I have done this". The sleeve arrived and was duly fitted. It was a tight fit and quite difficult to put on. Each night it was removed and fitted again the next morning. In spite of this, the swelling stubbornly refused to go down and Linda's mastectomy was scheduled for August 27th.

On August 11th the Haven was holding a "Laughter Workshop", which was open to all of their clients. Linda didn't feel up to going but I was intrigued by it and booked my place. It turned out to be an exhilarating experience taken by a laughter therapist, Margaret McCathie. She was a big, open hearted, wonderful person with a very special story to tell. She had been a successful therapist, who had fallen into serious depression. In her desperation she had contacted Patch Adams, who was featured in the Robin Williams movie of the same name. He advised her to start her journey to recovery by getting her eyes off herself and on to others. She followed his advice and recovered enough to visit Patch in America. He was so impressed with Margaret that he invited her on his world tour. He used a lot of humour when sensitively interacting with others. Margaret saw the benefit and became a laughter therapist. I was really impressed by her. So much of what she said resonated with what Linda and I were experiencing, that I arranged to see her for a wee chat.

Linda continued to get stronger as the date for her operation drew near. The only blemish on the landscape was her swollen arm, despite our best efforts with the sleeve.

We had not had a holiday that year and our neighbours Rhona and Norrie very kindly invited us to stay at their residential caravan on the west coast of Scotland at Maidens near Ayr. We gratefully accepted their offer and planned to go from August 17th – 21st. It would be a little treat for Linda, a week before her operation.

I had enjoyed caravan holidays when the kids were small but had been less keen on them as we got older, preferring the comfort of a holiday cottage or hotel. However, when we saw the lovely, spacious caravan, we rejoiced at the generosity of our dear neighbours. We had not brought much food with us so a wee exploration of our locality in the car followed. We earmarked restaurants to visit and picked one for the next day's lunch. It was with a spirit of thankfulness that we settled in for our first night. We looked forward the next day to leisurely walks, visits to nearby attractions and tasty food.

Next morning as Linda came out of the shower, she did something to her back and it went into spasm. She could hardly move and she had no alternative but to rest. We thought about going home, but it seemed such a shame and decided to persevere and make the best of it. As for our lunchtime plan it was obvious that Linda wasn't going to make it. I was dispatched to see if I could get a carryout somewhere. However as I left the caravan, I came up with the bright idea to visit the original selected restaurant, explain my predicament and see if they would give us a carryout. They were very understanding and supplied us with the tasty food. Back at the caravan Linda's face lit up at the sight of such lovely fare. We ate our lunches with thankful hearts.

As the day progressed, Linda's back pain eased. We spent most of that day admiring the lovely views of the Ayrshire coast from our caravan windows and reading books that we had brought with us. I bought some food and cooked an evening meal. The next day Linda's back was a bit better, but still prone to go into spasm. We tentatively explored the surrounding locality in the car, selecting only areas that were on the flat. Linda never had problems with her back before and sensibly rested a lot that day to allow her back to recover.

During the remaining two days, Linda's back gradually recovered and we were able to travel further afield. It was "Burns' Country" and we visited most of the attractions. Memories that stand out included visiting the lovely Brig o' Doon House Hotel, with a leisurely walk through the beautiful gardens to be followed by a splendid dinner; lunch at the Tam O'Shanter Teahouse and dinner at a lovely restaurant adjacent to the caravan site. We took lots of photos and really enjoyed ourselves. The morning of the 21st saw us packing up and returning home, feeling refreshed with thankful hearts.

On the 24th Linda had an afternoon appointment with Mr Murphy, three days before the date of her operation. I had an appointment to see Margaret McCathie at the same time, so I cancelled it and accompanied Linda. Her arm remained stubbornly swollen and Mr Murphy discussed with us whether or not to proceed with the operation. His recommendation was to carry on with the mastectomy and removal of the lymph nodes in her left arm. We trusted his judgement and agreed to go ahead.

Linda was so brave through all of this. She had a quiet confidence about her and all our dear friends gathered around us to give their support. We had developed an intimacy with so many people and at the end of each night, as we did our evening devotions, we felt abundantly blessed.

We felt really apprehensive when the day of the operation came. I transported Linda to Monklands hospital in Airdrie and intended to stay by her side as much as I could. During the booking-in process, we had a visit from the anaesthetist, who turned out to be another lovely woman. She went through each stage of the operation with us and explained what she was going to do. Linda had a number of questions and she was able to answer them all satisfactorily. She had such a confident manner about her and as she talked, I could see some of the tension drain from Linda. I thought that I would have to leave Linda at an early stage, but they let me stay with her right up until she was wheeled into the operating theatre.

The operation went very well and Linda recovered pretty quickly. Within a day she was sitting up in bed joking with us. She was sent home four days after the operation. Linda was worried about how she would feel with her breast missing. I reassured her that it would not make any difference to me. When she came home I had to help her shower and although I found it sad to see her this way, I was just so glad to have her with me again. She seemed to take it pretty well and was just pleased to be alive. We rejoiced that we had successfully nego-tiated two of the three hurdles, with only the radiotherapy left.

Chapter 5
Early September – Bad News

*M*y brother Dave had emigrated to Canada 40 years before and had become a very successful art dealer. Like us, he had three boys and our families were close. His wife Alison was a wonderful person and Linda just loved it when we all got together. They had been shocked by Linda's diagnosis and had been a terrific support as we journeyed together. Dave was the adventurer in the family and whenever we met he always told exciting stories about his exploits. He was also a very kind and extremely generous individual and I was proud to have him as my brother.

Their eldest son Alan had decided to get married at relatively short notice. It was to take place in Winnipeg on September 5th. We would have loved to go, but it was not possible, so we sent our youngest son Iain, as our family representative. Iain loved travelling and flew out on Thursday the 3rd to attend the celebrations.

The previous day Linda had attended Monklands for a bone scan. The procedure was non invasive and passed without any problems. An appointment for a CAT scan at the Golden Jubilee Hospital in Clydebank was scheduled for the 8th.

On Monday the 7th Linda had a "routine" appointment with Mr Murphy and we attended it with much optimism. Jackie, one of the breast care nurses whom we had grown to love and respect, was also in attendance. Our thoughts were about fixing a date for the radiotherapy and still being "clear by Christmas". His news devastated both of us.

The tissue samples obtained during the mastectomy had shown that the **cancer was still active in all her breast tissue and all the lymph nodes**. The only good news was that the bone scan, from the previous day, had shown no abnormalities. The planned CAT scan would reveal if the cancer had spread any further. We felt numb as we tried to take in what he said. Mr Murphy was such a kind and gracious man; we could tell that his heart went out to both of us. The tears ran down my beautiful Linda's face and I held her in my arms.

We had put ourselves into their hands, done everything that was asked of us and all the time the cancer had been spreading! We trusted them, they knew best and now this! It seemed that we had entered a new world as we struggled to adjust to the news. There was nothing else, surgically to be done. An appointment was scheduled with Dr Hicks on Tuesday the 15th to review our options. We recognised that Mr Murphy had done everything he could and in many instances, had *"gone the extra mile"* in attending to Linda. It appeared that he was withdrawing from our lives, redundant. We thanked him for all his kindness and expertise and we parted with sad hearts.

I telephoned a few close friends. They were as shocked as we were and pledged their continuing support. Linda and I decided that we were going to fight this with all of our resources and we recommitted ourselves into God's hands. We used the "Northumbrian Daily Office" book for our evening devotions and claimed the promise once more that "God had a plan for our lives, for good and not for evil".

Linda was a bit apprehensive about the CAT scan appointment the next day. Before the start of her chemotherapy Linda had undergone this test and they experienced difficulty getting a line into her arm. By now Linda's veins were in a very poor state and only the most experienced practitioner could carry this out. As was our practice, we had committed the whole situation to God but it was with much apprehension that Linda was taken for the procedure. After 30 minutes, she returned with a smile on her face. She had explained the difficulty to the radiography staff and they had called on the services of a medic who was very skilled in phlebotomy and who just "happened" to be on duty. The whole thing went very smoothly and we rejoiced together, thanking God for his provision. Little events like this had been and would continue to be, sources of encouragement, indicating that God was going before us, preparing the way.

News filtered through to Daniel Kish in the USA and he sent me a very challenging email. Among other qualifications, he was an educational psychologist and was very skilled at understanding people. He graciously shared his insight and when I read it, I recognised that he understood Linda. He said that she was one of the most wonderful people he had ever met. However, she liked to follow the safe, traditional paths. What was needed for this extraordinary situation was the courage to leave her comfort zone and try a new way. He suggested that we do not continue with the conventional treatment, but fly Linda out to the Hippocrates Institute in America for naturopathic treatment. I showed the E mail to Linda and she recognised herself in what Daniel had said. We decided to keep all of our options open.

It was with much trepidation that Linda and I attended the appointment with Dr Hicks on the following Tuesday (15th). Beforehand we had encouraged each other that at least the cancer had not spread to Linda's bones. We were so glad to see Jackie there too.

His news could not have been worse! Apart from her breast areas, the cancer had now also spread to Linda's liver and bones. Once again we were stunned! How could this be? We were used to finding something positive to cling on to, but there was not one encouraging thing in sight.

The talk was no longer about cures, but survival times. "If" we wanted to continue with treatment, the only option was more chemotherapy with an anti-bone cancer component added. There was a choice to be made, whether Linda continue or not, with no optimistic outcome for either. We could take our time about making the decision, even a few weeks. We asked for time to "get our heads around it" and went to the canteen for a cup of tea.

Dr Hicks had given us little grounds for hope. However to give up the fight seemed unthinkable. The cancer was continuing to spread, even as we talked. We returned to the department and were waiting to see Dr Hicks again when Jackie sat down beside us. She shared her concern with us, that the interview had seemed so devoid of hope. In her experience some patients, given the same prognosis, had survived for up to two years and a few had even lived up to five years. It was a really difficult journey and she wasn't trying to hide that from us, but it was possible. We felt encouraged and the faint spark of hope that we had, grew a little brighter. I commented that we would not be so passive this time, but be more challenging and be open to different alternatives.

We returned to see Dr Hicks and Linda informed him that she wished to continue with chemotherapy. A date was set for the following Tuesday to start her treatment. Her chemotherapy would include anti bone cancer agents. It was agreed that we could always change it if we came up with an alternative.

Iain had that day returned from the Canadian wedding and was at home to greet us. He was shocked by the news and held us close with one of his wonderful hugs. Linda was tired and went to bed. I phoned the rest of our family and friends with the terrible news. They were as shocked as we were and rallied round in support.

September was proving a difficult month. We continued with our routine of rising each morning and doing the morning "Northumbrian Office" liturgy. We would thank God for that day and commit it into His hands. "One day at a time" was one of our mottos.

I had read a book called "Tuesdays with Marnie" by Mitch Album. The author was visiting his old professor who was terminally ill. Each Tuesday, his professor would share little gems of wisdom with him. One such gem was that he would allow 20 minutes to feel sorry for himself each day and then get on with his life. We had found this attitude to be helpful on our journey and sought to continue practising it. After the allocated 20 minutes, we would hug each other and then try as best as we could to get on with life.

The prospect of Linda having to undergo another toxic round of chemotherapy did not inspire us, so I investigated alternatives. There was a plethora of treatments and philosophies all claiming efficacy. I decided to only consider those that came recommended by more than one source.

The Hippocrates Institute naturopathy philosophy, with its concentration on the raw food diet, was probably at the top of the list. There were a number of coincidences in our dealings with Daniel and Ram. They had both cast doubts on the chemotherapy regime from the start and questioned the principle of destroying Linda's own natural defence mechanisms in an attempt to eradicate the cancer. Ram had even prepared questions for us to ask our team.

However our strategy had been to keep it simple, not ask too many questions and just trust the experts. We had found them to be lovely, dedicated people and developed really close relationships with them. We could have delved in further, but we were scared enough as it was, with the little we had read. In fact a deliberate decision was made not to delve any further. I especially, was a consummate worrier and had struggled for years with what was termed a "generalised anxiety disorder". Linda had a simple faith and trusting nature. It was best to let God do the worrying and put our trust in Him and the experts. Perhaps this was a cop out, but it was what we had decided.

During Fraser and Larinda's visit in June, Linda and I had relaxed in the mornings by reading books. At the time I was being coached in the raw food diet by Ram, so I chose to read "The Live Food Factor", by Susan Schenck. Previously, every time I started reading a book, I tended to fall asleep after reading a few pages. However I found that I was able to read it, a section at a time and maintain my concentration. I had almost finished it, but had discontinued reading after Linda had "freaked out" over my weight loss. It certainly gave food for thought (pardon the pun), claiming drastic improvements in numerous diseases including cancer. The downside to it was that to be fully effective, the diet was vegan (vegetarian with no animal or fish products at all) with no cooked food, wheat or sugar. As I have already commented, Linda and I loved our food. In many ways we planned our lives around what and where we would eat. Did we "eat to live" or "live to eat"? The book termed this as an "addiction" to cooked food.

Another treatment which came to the fore advocated the consumption of crushed apricot kernels, which allegedly had anti-cancer properties. A centre in the USA claimed success in treating cancer with them. On checking out the contacts in the UK, we found that they were part of a praying Christian community who saw this as their "ministry" in the fight against cancer. Perhaps God was leading us to this! The downside was that to be effective in Linda's case, very high doses were needed. She would also need very expensive supplements. We considered this and ordered a supply of the kernels, just in case.

We also considered visiting a holistic practitioner, in nearby Dunblane, who claimed on her website to be able to help.

Chapter 6
September continued - An Encounter with the Laughter Therapist

After the ill-fated meeting with Mr Murphy, I had a persistent feeling that Linda would benefit from meeting Margaret, the Laughter Therapist. I had originally wanted to see her for myself to help me on *my journey*, but this was to be about helping Linda in *her journey*. We discussed it together and she readily agreed to see Margaret if that were possible. A couple of days later, on Friday September 18th, we drove into Bridge of Allan, a picturesque village about an hour's drive from our home in Blantyre. Linda had never been in the village before and was enchanted by it. As we searched for Margaret's house, we promised ourselves that after we had met with Margaret, we would go exploring.

Margaret gave us a lovely welcome at the door of her wonderful, big house. Linda took to her straight away and soon they were chatting like long lost friends. I stood back in wonder as I saw two really special people getting to know one another.

Margaret shared some of her background with Linda. One of the reasons she had fallen into serious depression was that she had a deep need for the approval of others. She had spent most of her life motivated by this, at a serious cost to her mental health. One outcome was that she always thought her husband would leave her. When recovering from her illness, this underground driving force came to the fore. Margaret was able to acknowledge it and let it go. This insight had been crucial in her road to recovery and she now had a much freer relationship with people in general and her husband in particular.

As Linda listened, she identified this same deep seated need for approval in her own life and she shared her experience of this with Margaret. She had also feared that I would leave her. As she shared, something seemed to shift in Linda's psyche and miraculously, she was able to shed this burden. I stood by and watched the process in wonder. Linda expressed a number of emotions, from sadness at her lifetime's waste of energy in trying to satisfy this need, to joy at her feelings of release. I felt privileged to be there and now understood why I needed to arrange this meeting.

As if that was not enough, something was happening to me simultaneously, at the edge of my awareness. I was recognising this same driving force in my own life. In particular I was aware of my deep need for approval from the opposite sex. However, I was conscious that this meeting was about Linda and refocused my attention on what was happening to her.

We discussed alternative treatments with Margaret. She believed in the efficacy of apricot kernels and her husband took them each morning with his breakfast. His PSA test result for prostate cancer had been positive but had returned to normal.

I had been seriously considering the Hippocrates Institute option and so I explained to her about receiving Daniel's email. Margaret listened with interest and I offered it to her to read. She decided that a break for a cup of tea was necessary and retired to the kitchen, clutching the email.

Left alone together, we began to share what was happening in each of us. We shared the impact on our lives trying to satisfy our common, deep seated need for approval. I felt really close to Linda as I shared my deep need for approval of others and in particular with the opposite sex. Linda had interpreted this as a mark of dissatisfaction with her and was able to see it in a new light. Then she said tenderly, "If I don't make it through this, it's OK to marry someone else". Our hearts were open to each other; tears flowed as we embraced.

After a few minutes Margaret returned with a lovely spread of tea and scones. She had read Daniel's email and was taken with the clarity of his insight. Margaret expressed a strong intuitive sense that this was for Linda. We discussed it further and I also expressed my sense that this may be the way forward. Linda did not say much and just listened. It had been a rich time for all of us and we parted with thankful hearts.

Remembering our promised exploration, we drove back into the centre of the village and parked the car. We then took our time to meander through it, appreciating all the sights, smells and people. There seemed to me a clarity and freshness about everything and a sense of timelessness. We realised we were hungry and eventually found a lovely restaurant for a late lunch.

Our openness with each other was very special and I shared another area of my life, which I felt had been influenced by my need for approval. Linda had always been puzzled by my attitude to her mother. She saw me being kind and considerate to almost everyone else, but detected an impatience and antagonism to her mum. I did lots of things for her, but there was resentment there and it came to the fore with an occasional scathing comment. We had discussed it openly together and I had admitted that Linda was spot on with her assessment. My explanation for my behaviour was that, somehow I didn't "take" to her mum and I defended myself, that I could not be expected to "take" to everyone. However my explanation had never sat well with me, or with Linda.

I now sensed that my need for approval was also at the heart of this and as it came to the fore, it did not show me in a good light. I did not rate Linda's mum as an important person and basically she was getting in the way of my subconscious, life-long search for approval. The many things I did for her I did out of a sense of duty, not love and mainly to be seen by others. My acting out of this scenario was not able to be maintained all the time, hence my scathing comments. I now sensed that something in me had shifted in my relationship with Linda's mum (Margaret).

This shift became evident in the next few days. I found I now had an open heart to Linda's mum and was able to love her for herself, with no strings attached. Linda noticed my new, kind attitude to her mum and I remember her questioning me. My response was that simply my heart had been changed and now I loved her mum. I viewed my past behaviour with regret and sadness, but I could not change the past. Linda expressed her incredulity at this difference in me. She had always felt extremely uncomfortable about the relationship and had continually felt torn between conflicting loyalties. Another burden had been lifted from her and she was so thankful. As for myself, I experienced clearly the difference between doing something out of love and doing something out of duty.

Over the next few days we both independently noticed another wonderful difference. Linda's mum seemed to change in subtle ways. She seemed to "blossom" somehow, was more accepting and less liable to complain (she had always found something to complain about). We attributed this change to be her subconscious response to the difference in my attitude and we stood back in wonder. There appeared to be a ripple effect from the visit to the laughter therapist.

It is worth noting that I was learning some wonderful lessons on our journey together. I found myself using my background in the counselling profession to seek to understand the underlying principles.

When I consciously took my eyes off myself and my needs, and placed them on the needs of "the other", without judgement, I was able to see their "beauty". This met their need to be understood and appreciated. They responded to being met in this way, by reciprocating the process and seeing my "*beauty*" and meeting some of my needs. Both parties ended up being enriched by the process. Put it another way, when I consciously made the meeting be about the other and not me, wonderfully it became about the other **and** me.

I was also learning to appreciate the "Grace of God". If I continually take my eyes off myself and on to others and use this as a formula for living, it will probably be a good thing to do. However, add a reverence for the "Grace of God" to the process and wonderful things can happen. When I appreciate that all I am doing is opening my heart to the "other" and leaving space for God's "Grace" to work, that is reflected in my attitude. I am filled with a sense of wonder and it stops me from thinking that "I"did it.

My understanding about this deep need for approval was that it didn't just disappear in either of our lives. Perhaps it is there in most of our lives, as it is a perfectly normal need. The problem arises when it exerts undue influence. It simply loosened its grip on us. Hopefully, now that it was more out in the open, we were able to recognise its influence and be freer to make choices as to our behaviour.

Chapter 7
September Continued - Hippocrates Institute

After our eventful meeting with the Laughter Therapist, I was becoming convinced that God was leading me to take Linda to the Hippocrates Institute for treatment. After all, we both had the promise from God's word that He had a plan for Linda's life, "for good and not for evil".

I took the initiative and did a number of things. First I looked into the practicalities of doing this. I contacted the Institute and found out the cost and availability for both of us to go. Then I looked at travel insurance. Money was not important. Whatever the cost, if Linda decided to go, we would go.

I contacted Stuart, Fraser and Dave and sent them Daniel's email, explaining what we were considering.

Dave was the first to respond. A lot of his wonderful stories happened because he trusted his gut feeling. He felt that same feeling now about Linda attending the Institute. *"Go with it"* he advised.

Stuart lived in Lagrange, Georgia, which was relatively close (a few hundred miles) to the Institute. I asked him to find out what he could about their work and reputation. Replies came back. Jessica had visited the website and in her opinion, "it was just a glorified Spa". Stuart was a little more open to the possibility and felt that if we decided to take Linda there, he would support our decision. Jessica's mum was a lovely lady. She was a part-time Methodist minister and I respected her judgement. Since she lived in the same general area, I was hopeful that she would have had some contact with the Institute, or would know of their work. She replied that she had no knowledge of them.

Fraser in Canada had had a fair amount of contact with Daniel over the years. After some consideration he replied that he was in favour of the Hippocrates option. Iain, back home, also approved.

I also contacted Steve, Linda's minister and asked him to pray for God's guidance. Perhaps God would give Steve a "sign". Steve replied that he was not happy about doing that and I sensed that he was not in favour of the trip.

After all the information had been collected I presented it to Linda. It seemed that the majority of her supporters were in favour. There was a choice to be made between more chemotherapy and the Institute. The first appointment for the new chemotherapy regime was a few days away, on September 22nd. Alternatively she could be in the USA for treatment within a week. I confess that I was not neutral and really wanted her to go because I thought that was where God was leading us. I also saw what the chemotherapy did to her and was not keen for her to go through an even worse experience.

Linda was not so sure and expressed anxiety about leaving the security of her home and travelling halfway around the world, away from all her support. What if she became unwell? However for me, Daniel's challenge came to the fore. "Linda liked to follow the safe, traditional paths. What was needed for this extraordinary situation was the courage to leave her comfort zone and try a new way". Linda continued to be troubled, struggling with the need to make a decision amid the different pressures placed on her.

Eventually she indicated that she had made the decision and we sat down together. She had decided to stay with the conventional treatment and tearfully apologised to me for not having the courage to follow Daniel's advice. She expressed regret that she had "failed me", hence her apology. Her words pierced my heart! Linda had shown tremendous courage all through this journey. She could never fail me! How dare I put pressure on her to do what I wanted? My heart went out to her and I felt really bad about the way I had treated her. I reassured her that I respected her decision and would support her wholeheartedly.

Linda's face lit up and I could see the burden being lifted from her. I loved her with every ounce of my being. We held each other and shed tears of joy together. The Hippocrates option was finished with and would not be mentioned again. It was great to feel this unity again and we could now gather our combined strengths to face the fresh challenges ahead. I felt suitably chastised by this experience, recognising the necessity of taking my leading from Linda and not getting carried away with my enthusiasm.

I contacted Daniel and Ram, expressing my thanks for their concern and informing them of Linda's decision. They replied with understanding emails and wished us well. The family members involved also pledged their continuing support.

Chapter 8
Late September / Early October - Stuart's Visit;

Stuart in the USA decided that he would visit us for a week starting on September 29th. We were looking forward to seeing him as we had visited them in August 2008 and had rejoiced in getting to know our new granddaughter Norah, who was then only two months old. She was such a beautiful baby and Linda just loved every minute of our visit. Linda had a special gift when it came to relating to children and it was a joy seeing them together. We also treasured Jessica as a daughter-in-law and in our short time together we felt a real closeness. It would have been great to for us to see the whole family again, but that was not possible. It was a wonderful surprise therefore, when Stuart phoned us to say they were all coming.

Our lives were full of so many encouragements as we gathered up our resources to face the battle ahead. On September 22nd we attended Wishaw General for the start of the new chemotherapy regime. The staff were really kind, but I felt there was a subtle change in their attitude. I thought I detected a sadness in their manner, which was not there before. There was no talk of the future anymore, but there was a sense of their deep caring. The chemotherapy was administered without incident and we returned home with thankful hearts. Linda had a week to recover and then Stuart and his family would be here.

I was still looking for more natural, less toxic ways to fight her illness and I considered the administration of crushed apricot kernels to augment her chemotherapy. I contacted Jackie and asked if that would be possible. She checked with the hospital pharmacist, who gave us some literature, which questioned the claims of efficacy. However, she said that if we wanted to add the kernels to the regime, they would respect our wishes and it should not affect the conventional agents.

I gathered all the information that I had on the subject and took it to Linda. She could begin with small doses and then see how it went. There was an acknowledgement that to have any significant effect, pretty large doses would be required. Linda was hesitant and this time I respected her feelings. All these conventional toxic substances in her system and then adding something else, which potentially could also be toxic! I left Linda to consider what she wanted to do.

Given the previous experience of my enthusiasm to find a less toxic way ahead, I reflected on what I was doing. I was always very apprehensive when it came to taking any medication myself, fearing the side effects. Here I was, asking my beloved to do something, which I probably would not have the courage to do myself. I shared this with Linda and she smiled with relief. She didn't really want to go on the kernels and was not looking forward to telling me. It was another salutary lesson and I saw clearly that my role was to support Linda in whatever road she chose. She was the brave one and had shown tremendous courage throughout. I experienced a peace about the way ahead and stopped searching for alternative "magical" cures.

On September 29th Stuart arrived with his family. Linda remained at home while I met them at the airport. It was great to see them and we spent such precious times together. Wee Norah was an angel and Linda just loved her to bits. She was able to do all the normal things with her i.e. giving her a bath, feeding her and getting her ready for bed. We didn't travel too far, but we didn't have to, since so many of our favourite places such as the nearby park, Bothwell Castle and the loch at the heritage park in East Kilbride were close by. Fortunately the weather was pretty good and we were so thankful. Everyone wanted to see Stuart, Jessica and Norah and our house was busy with visitors. Great Gran (Linda's mum) was a regular visitor, while Malcolm and Margaret (Linda's brother and sister-in-law), Billy and Cathy (Linda's uncle and aunt) all visited. It was also a joy to attend the Sunday morning service in Linda's church. Jessica was known to them, in that she had visited Scotland twice previously, but of course none of them had met Norah. It was great for them to meet the "wee stunner" in the flesh. We were blessed with having so many special friends in the church and it was great to have fellowship together.

Stuart remembers

"Norah at that age was always very shy when meeting people and it would take a couple of days before she would play with them. However Norah took immediately to mum, giving her hugs and playing with her. I remember mum taking her to the park and having fun with her on the swings. Norah laughed with pleasure the whole time. I also have a picture in my mind of mum and her sharing an ice cream at Bothwell Castle. Mum loved especially the curls in Norah's hair and was very adept at getting onto Norah's level."

Jessica remembers.

"Linda was always taking care of everybody in a very quiet and motherly way. During this trip however I had the wonderful experience of giving Linda a manicure, pedicure and hand massage. I loved caring for her in this way.

Linda was still carrying on as normal as possible with cleaning and cooking, but this trip was different somehow. When I offered to do the dishes, she agreed so that she could play with Nora or rest. I felt that this was a gift from her – to allow me to take the maternal role. How simple life was that week – a loving family, loving God, no TV, no commotion, work etc. We were able to focus on what was important."

Both Stuart and Jessica remember especially the evening devotions together as being beautiful and unique experiences, which they will always treasure. Jessica recalls us all being in tears at the end one time. Stuart was very taken by our simple philosophy, *"taking our eyes off ourselves and onto others"* He also remembers thanking his mum for the person she was and how she had shaped his life. Alas, the time sped by and on October 6th we said our tearful goodbyes. We consoled ourselves with the hope of visiting them when Linda finished this round of chemotherapy.

Chapter 9
Early October – Healing Option & Further Bad News

*L*ife returned to "normal" after Stuart's visit. Needless to say Linda was pretty tired after all the excitement. She loved aromatherapy and had accepted the Haven's offer of weekly sessions, attending the first one on Thursday October 8th. Linda did a small amount of baking for her church's coffee morning on the following Saturday.

The next day at my church, I had an interesting conversation with a retired Episcopal minister friend called Aiden. He was a very warm, loving man and I had grown quite close to him and his wife, Sarah. They had prayerfully supported us throughout Linda's journey. After the service, over coffee, he asked if we had ever thought about the ministry of healing. He had attended the King's Centre in nearby Motherwell, where they practised this. People had testified of receiving remarkable healings from God.

Linda and I had discussed the ministry of healing earlier in her illness, but at that time she wanted to concentrate on conventional treatment. When I got home from church, I related my conversation with Aiden to her and asked her if she was open to going down that way. Perhaps God had sent Aiden to us and this was part of His plan for our lives. She indicated that she was now open to the possibility and asked me to make further enquiries. I contacted Aiden and he gave me the contact name of Rev David Currie.

Linda's second chemotherapy session was looming on Tuesday the 13th. She was pretty tired, so I borrowed a wheelchair (which previously had been my dad's and I had gifted to the Baptist church) to conserve her energy. We attended it with much trepidation. The session began with blood samples being taken by the expert nurses. They had always got them at the first attempt but this time it took two or three. Linda's veins were deteriorating fast! Next on the schedule was a meeting with Dr Hicks to assess Linda's condition before sanctioning another round of chemotherapy. There was a delay before we were called in to see Dr Hicks. When he eventually called us, he gave us the news that the next round of chemotherapy had to be postponed. Linda's blood tests had shown that she was very anaemic and had a low platelet count (platelets are needed to help stop bleeding). Arrangements were made for her to attend Monklands hospital that afternoon for a blood transfusion. He encouraged us by saying that the next round of chemotherapy should be only delayed for a week.

We were pretty shocked by this turn of events but consoled ourselves by remembering the very first round of chemotherapy. It had started off with her allergic reaction and she still managed to complete the course. Once again we committed ourselves into God's hands. Linda was very tired when we arrived home and after lunch she went for a wee nap, as there was time before we needed to go to Monklands.

That afternoon Linda was admitted to ward 6 for the blood transfusion. It did not start well. The junior medic could not get a central line in. After she tried two or three times I was getting very concerned and gently suggested she get help. As it happened, Jackie, the breast control nurse, was in the department. She skilfully got the line in first time.

We thanked God for sending her to help us. The transfusion went smoothly and we returned home.

After the transfusion, Linda seemed to perk up a bit and she attended her weekly aromatherapy session on Friday 15th. We spent a quiet weekend together and appreciated each other's company after our busy schedule with Stuart and his family. She wanted a new wig and had arranged a Monday appointment to see Marion at the Haven. Marion was such a wonderful person and Linda loved to see her. It was a nice preparation for the next day's rescheduled chemotherapy appointment.

In the morning Linda's energy levels were really low so I used the wheelchair again to transport her from the car to the chemotherapy unit. As was our practice, we had committed the whole day to God and were resting in His hands.

Once again, they had trouble getting blood from Linda, but were eventually successful. While we waited patiently to see Dr Hicks, I noticed that she had fallen asleep in the wheelchair. I admired Linda's trusting spirit.

When Dr Hicks eventually called us in we were glad to also see Jackie in attendance. It seemed that recently he had given us nothing but bad news; surely this session would be different! Nothing could have prepared us for his assessment.

It appeared that Linda's cancer had spread even further. The planned chemotherapy was no longer viable. There was nothing they could offer her! Her platelet count was dangerously low, but it was pointless giving her a platelet transfusion, as the transfused platelets would only last a few days in her system. He advised us not to call the emergency services if Linda became unwell at home. They would just admit her to hospital and subject her to unnecessary trauma.

We were shocked by the gravity of his assessment and I struggled to take it in. It sounded to me that they were sending her home to die! Linda appeared to be in a state of shock as she tried to process what she had been told. I gathered myself together and asked Dr Hicks how long my beloved Linda had left. He turned to face Linda. He gently explained that he did not answer that question when a relative asked it, but if she wanted to know his assessment, he would give it to her. After a few minutes she whispered, "No, I don't want to know".

My heart went out to her and we held each other's hands. I repeated Dr Hick's assessment back to him, just to clarify that I understood what we were supposed to do if Linda was unwell. I commented to Dr Hicks, that perhaps one day, he would be able to give us good news again. He seemed taken aback when I asked about the date for the next appointment, but gave us one for three weeks ahead. On leaving I commented to Linda that we would prove him wrong. We would find a way through this and see him again. There would be good news again!

We were both in a daze as we travelled home in silence. This was interrupted by a call on my mobile phone from Jackie. They had reconsidered and had decided to transfuse Linda with platelets. We were to attend Monklands that afternoon for the transfusion. I felt encouraged. Perhaps they had not given up hope either.

Chapter 10
October continued - The Platelet Transfusion

*A*fter lunch Linda went for a wee nap in preparation for her platelet transfusion. Meanwhile I phoned a few of our close supporters and updated them. They were grieved by the news and promised to continue in prayer. I also contacted the Rev David Currie at the King's Centre and arranged for Linda and I to attend their healing meeting next day, Wednesday 21st at 11am. I was determined that no stone would be left unturned as we sought a way through.

Linda was admitted into ward 6 and we were pleased to see Jackie in attendance again. The platelets were ready for us and Jackie prepared to insert a line into Linda's arm. She tried three times, but to our dismay, failed each time.

"Oh, bugger it," she said in frustration. "I am not going to be able to do this. It's pointless me trying again. I'll need to see if I can get someone else to try."

This shouldn't be happening, I thought in despair. *If Jackie can't do it, nobody can!*

The junior medic was also in attendance. "I'll give it a try," she offered and started to make preparations.

I felt really uncomfortable as I recognised her as the same medic who had been unsuccessful in taking a routine blood sample prior to Linda's blood transfusion the week before.

I looked Jackie in the eye.

"I want you to try one more time. I feel that you are the person who can do this. Try it again and if you are unsuccessful, we will give up".

Jackie gave a wry smile. "No pressure then!"

I seemed to get the confidence and knowledge from somewhere that this was the right thing to do and Jackie steeled herself for one more attempt. Imagine our joy when Jackie was successful. We all expressed a collective sigh of relief and rejoiced together. I thanked God for his provision.

As I sat by Linda's bedside and watched the platelets being transfused, my mind kept on going over the implications of what Dr Hicks had said. Linda and I had not really talked about it and I respected her wish not to know about timescales. I gently reiterated what he had said to her and tentatively asked.

'Linda, do you understand?"

She regarded me with sadness in her eyes, nodded her head and drifted off to sleep.

I had a need to know what we were facing. There was a way through this, but I needed to talk to someone with the knowledge, so I could prepare myself. Jackie was still in the ward, so I sought her out and asked if we could talk. I explained that although Linda did not want to know about timescales, my need was different.

"I want to know if Linda's time left is in; hours; days; weeks; months or years".

She pondered for a moment before giving her reply. "It may be hours or days, perhaps even weeks, but it is unlikely to be longer than that".

My heart sank because this was what I suspected. Tears ran down my cheeks and Jackie comforted me by giving me a wonderful hug. I composed myself, thanked her for her candour and returned to Linda's bedside.

As I sat by her bedside again I uttered a desperate prayer. "We believed that You had a plan for our lives, for good and not for evil, to give us hope and a good future. What now God?"

The incident with the insertion of lines had shown it. *What was His plan?* My thoughts turned to the next day's' healing meeting. Perhaps God would heal my beloved. I resolved to take Linda there. After the transfusion was finished, I transferred Linda to her wheelchair, thanked everyone and walked towards the lift.

The lift doors opened and we came face to face with the surgeon, Mr Murphy. We were surprised as we never expected to see him again. He had a sadness in his eyes and I realised that he knew our situation.

"I cannot tell you how sorry I am. How are you both doing?"

We had heard that he was a committed Christian and I felt that he would understand, so I explained.

"We are not giving up. I am taking Linda to a Christian healing meeting tomorrow."

He smiled and, shaking our hands, said, "God bless you both".

Although it had been a very testing day, I felt God's provision and was encouraged by this chance meeting. Perhaps another "angel" had been sent to help us on our journey.

Chapter 11
Tuesday Evening October 20th – Back Home

Linda was exhausted when we returned home after the platelet transfusion and I helped her into bed. She fell asleep immediately. Local nurses phoned to say that they had been notified of Linda's condition and would be visiting us shortly. I jotted down all the things that I had to do and set about doing them.

I phoned Stuart in the USA and Fraser in Canada and explained the gravity of the situation to them. Both promised to catch the next available flight home. My brother Dave in Canada was also contacted and he gave a similar commitment. I then rang Linda's brother Malcolm, who was a mail delivery driver. He was in the middle of his schedule and was shocked by the news. He phoned me back to say that he had terminated his run and would be with us as soon as possible. I also informed Linda's mum and a few close friends.

The local nurses arrived and set about administering the pain medication which would help Linda through the night. Macmillan nurses would attend the next day. They were the experts when it came to relieving pain and would probably set up a morphine syringe. Malcolm, Margaret and Linda's mum arrived and we comforted each other. As I regarded Linda's condition, I realised that she would be unable to attend the healing meeting. It was my last hope and I was not willing to give up on it. I contacted Rev David Currie and informed him that even if Linda was not able to attend, if possible I intended go in her place.

As midnight approached, there was nothing more to be done and everyone left, leaving Iain and I to care for her. Malcolm, Margaret and Linda's mum would be back the next morning. Iain reluctantly went to bed and I promised that I would wake him if needed.

It was a difficult night for Linda as she drifted in and out of consciousness. She was also wheezing a bit, which added to her discomfort. As I tended to her needs, I was aware of just how much I loved her and I counted it a privilege to care for my beloved in this way. However I was not giving up hope. Despite everything "God had a plan" and I still believed that it was possible that He would heal her.

Chapter 12
Wednesday, October 21st

*I*t was a busy house on the Wednesday morning. Nurses from the local health centre arrived to check Linda's condition. She had deteriorated a bit and they promised that Macmillan nurses would attend her later that day to install the morphine syringe. Hopefully she would not have to endure the discomfort of the previous night again.

The healing meeting at the King's Centre was from 11am to noon. I wanted to stay with Linda, but I was determined to go and fight for her life. Malcolm, Margaret and Linda's mum arrived and as Iain was also there, I left her in their capable hands. My mobile phone remained switched on so they could contact me at any time.

I was met at the King's Centre by David Black, who was a lovely, gracious, caring man. He shared his wonderful story of how he believed God had intervened and healed him of cancer. I had no reason to doubt him as he seemed a normal, balanced individual. He went on to introduce me to others who also claimed healing. I knew one of the couples and experienced a little disquiet about the authenticity of their claims.

I wondered *What am I getting myself into here?* However I was desperate and decided to see it through. After all, what harm could it do?

David explained the format of the meeting to me. Those leading the meeting stood on a platform and details of requests for prayers and answers to prayer would be announced by them. After highlighting all the requests for prayer, there would then be an open time of prayer. He turned to me and asked, "Would you be willing to stand in front of the meeting and personally introduce Linda and her situation to those present?" I readily agreed.

After the opening devotions, various people introduced loved ones' struggles and requested prayer for them. When it came to my turn, I stood on the platform and opened my heart to them. Tears streamed down my face as I explained my life and death struggle for my beloved Linda. An open time for prayer followed and various people came and prayed with me, some of them laying their hands on my head in the process. I was a little uncomfortable at the language used by some people.

"We bind the evil of the cancer in Jesus' name."

"We resist Satan in the name of Jesus and command him to leave Linda."

I deliberately put aside my disquiet. I did not care what descriptive terms they used. If it resulted in Linda's healing it was a price worth paying. I recognised that they were doing this out of love and they regarded this as their ministry. Perhaps it was me that had to change my understanding and God was leading me along this path.

When the meeting finished, I approached the leaders.

"Would it be possible for someone to visit Linda personally and pray for her healing?"

After discussion, a lady's voice piped up.

"I would be more than happy to come and visit Linda and pray with her".

"Me too", said her friend.

I was pleased with this, as I sensed the love in their hearts and returned home feeling satisfied that I had done everything I could.

I spent a lot of that day just sitting at her bedside, holding her hand and attending to her needs. She was beautiful and

I loved her so much. She wasn't really able to acknowledge me very much. However there was something that she was able to acknowledge and it was frozen packets of juice called Jubblies. When she drifted back into consciousness, she had a tremendous thirst and we would put a frozen Jubbly to her lips. Her face would light up in an ecstatic smile as she satisfied her thirst before drifting back into unconsciousness.

We all noticed this and I jokingly remarked, "Linda loves that Jubbly more than all of us put together".

However as the day passed into the evening, I felt myself becoming more unsettled and agitated. The reality was that the only thing she was able to acknowledge was the Jubbly. How I longed for her to acknowledge me in this last stage of her journey. My agitation became worse when I heard Gran, Malcolm and Margaret in the kitchen eating a meal and laughing together. I felt really angry. I stormed into the kitchen.

"How can you joke and enjoy a meal, with Linda dying next door?"

Thankfully they were able to acknowledge my anger and gathered round to support me with hugs and reassurance. In a strange way, somehow I seemed to feel secure enough in their love for me, to know that they would be able to hear my anger and not be offended.

I knew that I needed to go out for a walk to clear my head and so I left them to care for Linda. I walked 50 yards up our road and a lady who recognised me, asked why I did not have my dog with me. I was stunned. My wife was dying and I was looking for space to try to sort myself out and she was trying to have a normal conversation with me about dogs. I burst into tears and carried on past her.

However God sent me another couple of "angels" to help me through. The first one was a friend, an 80-year-old lady called Alice. She happened to be at her door and saw my reaction to the lady. She knew something of my situation and came running out and threw her arms around me to comfort me.

I really appreciated that hug. It was just what I needed and I thanked her for the practical demonstration of her care for me. I walked another 50 yards to pass the Baptist church. The second *"angel"* was the Baptist pastor Steve, who was a close friend. He was be standing at the church door and he could see that I was looking a bit dazed, so he called me over. I shared some of my struggles with him and he encouraged and comforted me. What were the chances of both of these people being on hand to minister to me in my need?

By the time I returned back home, I felt a lot better and resumed my duties at Linda's bedside. It was late evening and Gran, Malcolm and Margaret left to return to their respective homes, saying that they would come back in the morning.

Linda was having some difficulty breathing, so I called an emergency doctor. He arrived quickly and examined her. He detected fluid in her lungs and wanted her admitted to hospital. The advice from the oncologist rang in my ears, *"Don't let her be admitted to hospital. There is nothing that can be done for her and she will be subjected to unnecessary tests and trauma"*. I explained this to the emergency doctor. After a phone call to our GP, a compromise was reached and an oxygen cylinder was obtained to assist Linda in her breathing.

Nurses arrived and tried to show us the best way to adjust her position. Even although Linda was small, she was a dead weight and even they were having difficulty. I stood back at first, thinking that they would know best. They placed a plastic sheet underneath Linda and they had been trying to slide her up it toward the top of the bed. Eventually I intervened and showed them the method I had learned when I cared for my elderly father. It involved placing the plastic sheet under Linda and moving the sheet, instead of trying to move her. We tried it and it was much better. I could see that they were looking at me with a little more respect.

However this unsettled me a bit. If I was giving advice to the experts, had I done the right thing, trying to care for her at home? I had drawn on my experience to solve this problem. What would happen if another situation arose, where I did not have the experience? In hospital they had adjustable beds and other equipment that would certainly help in this situation. I phoned my friend Lachlan, an experienced nurse, and shared my concerns about my adequacy to be able to cope and give Linda the care she deserved. He offered to come up from Dumfries the next morning and help me with her care. I accepted his offer and felt reassured, thanking God once again for giving me so many wonderful friends.

Eventually Iain and I were left to look after her during the night. He brought his bed downstairs to just outside our room. I thanked God for the pillar of strength that my youngest son was turning out to be. Linda would sleep for 30 minutes at a time and then waken up. We would position her to raise her chest allowing her to breathe more easily and then we would administer the Jubbly. Her face would light up again for that moment and then she would drift back into unconsciousness.

As the night progressed, I began to feel unsettled again and believe it or not, a little jealous of the attention the Jubbly was receiving.

"Oh Linda my love, why can't you acknowledge me?" I pleaded from my heart.

Suddenly I realised what was happening. The awareness rushed in and I realised that I was feeling sorry for myself. I knew what I needed to do. I just simply took my eyes off myself for a moment and placed them on my beloved Linda again. What a difference! I felt an instantaneous release and my love for her flowed again. When she wakened, I manipulated her position to assist her breathing and gave her the Jubbly. Oh the joy that was in her face. When I saw her joy, my joy bubbled up from within me and I thanked God for this period of grace and revelation. I was on cloud nine for the remainder of the night, feeling really privileged to be able to care for her in this way.

Chapter 13
Thursday October 22nd

When morning came Lachlan arrived and I was thankful for his presence. He assessed her medical condition and gently stated: "Jim, Linda's body systems are gradually shutting down. You need to prepare yourself. She is unlikely to survive another day!"

As I struggled to adjust to this new timescale, my thoughts turned to our sons, Stuart and Fraser. They were rushing home to be with their mum and to say goodbye. Their flights would not arrive until the next day at the earliest. The realisation gradually dawned on me; they were probably going to be too late!

I felt so sad for them and imagined them arriving at Glasgow Airport to be told the news. *No way!* I thought. I contacted both of them and set up times later on in the day, when they could call their mum and say their goodbyes. Even although Linda was drifting in and out of consciousness and not able to visibly acknowledge us, I believed that she could hear us, as hearing is the last of the senses to go.

It was a busy time in the house with family and friends drifting in and out. The Macmillan nurses arrived to connect the morphine syringe. Local nurses were also in attendance. In the middle of all this the two ladies from the King's Centre arrived to administer their healing ministry. I explained to the nurses that I had not given up hope and they agreed to allow the ladies to pray for Linda at the same time. I found it a bit of a surreal experience, seeing them work side by side. Nurses attending to her physical needs and the ladies, "binding the evil of the cancer in the name of Jesus and demanding it leave her body". If the nurses found it strange, they did not show it. As for myself, I was open to whatever happened and was still clinging on to the hope that God would heal her.

The ladies finished and I thanked them for their ministry, recognising the love in their hearts.

Things settled down a bit and I resumed my bedside vigil, with the others sitting with me and giving me a break from time to time. As I regarded my beloved's gradual deterioration, Lachlan explained what was happening; I started to face up to the reality.

Linda was not going to be healed!

I had done all I could on this front, so I simply committed her into God's loving hands to do whatever He willed.

Stuart and Fraser phoned their mum for the last time and were able to tell her how much they loved her and say their goodbyes. It was a beautiful moment. Fraser reported told me later, "When I was saying my goodbyes to mum, her breathing changed, from being laboured at first, to becoming more relaxed, after our 'conversation.'"

I began to realise that I still had an expectation that during her last hours, she and I would be able to share our love for each other and say our goodbyes. I had seen it in the movies so many times, beautiful scenes with music playing in the background. I found myself reluctantly letting go of that dream and acknowledging the painful reality.

I would have preferred it to be different, but I realised that the drugs that controlled her pain also seemed to cut her off from me. I also remembered Linda's voice on previous occasions when we discussed death.

"When I die, I don't want to have it drawn out with a lot of suffering".

I continued to console myself with the hope that she could still hear me - even if there seemed to be no visible signs.

Although I felt Linda was cut off from me, something happened in the morning which showed that this was not the case. Linda was having trouble breathing and we constantly adjusted her position to raise her chest. Even with the technique with the plastic sheet it was an awkward process, causing Linda discomfort. I experimented climbing into her bed behind her, so that I might be able to achieve more leverage. This seemed to help and one of the times Lachlan climbed in behind her. Linda reacted immediately saying, "No! No!" leaving me in no doubt that she did not want Lachlan in the bed beside her. It was only two years later, when I was reflecting on this event, that I realised the significance of this. She was aware of what she wanted and what she did not want. When this was thwarted, she was aware enough to say so.

As the day progressed, Linda's condition continued to deteriorate. There was an acceptance from us all that it was now only a matter of time and I experienced a peace about the situation. Apart from those already mentioned, various really close friends dropped by wanting to spend time sitting with Linda and saying their goodbyes. They included Rhona, our next door neighbour, Jeanette and Myra from her work and Ann Cook, whom we had known and loved for years. I remember being surprised at how natural all this was and how all concerned added to the preciousness of the situation. I felt no resentment for the intrusions and gave thanks to God once again for giving us so many wonderful friends and family members.

During the last few hours of Linda's life, it was mainly Iain and I who sat at her bedside. We held a hand each and told her how much we loved her. It was a special time for us both, as we bonded even closer to her and to each other. Her breathing became more laboured and fitful as she slipped further into the coma. I remembered willing her to go and telling her that it was OK. A few times I thought that she had stopped breathing, only for her to start again, shallowly. Eventually she passed away peacefully and all was still. The time of death was 4.40pm.

Iain and I wept together. We informed family members and friends who were present in the house and they came to pay their last respects.

There were a number of tasks to be done now. I phoned the local health centre and a locum GP arrived. A month previously I had met her by chance and had been impressed by her respectful attitude. She very gently examined Linda and issued a death certificate. The undertaker was contacted and we made arrangements for Linda's body to be taken to their chapel. I telephoned all of the absent family members and a few close friends. I needed to be busy, to do everything I could to look as if I was coping and help me get through those first few hours without feeling sorry for myself.

I remember going in and out of the room every 10 minutes or so, holding her hand and gently kissing her lips, telling her how much I loved her and how beautiful she was. At first her body was still warm, but as time passed it became colder.

I received comfort from various neighbours coming into the house, spending a few moments sitting quietly beside her body and then silently leaving.

It was a strangely beautiful scene.

Chapter 14
Friday - Sunday, October 23rd - 25th – Initial Preparations for Funeral

The undertaker arrived later in the evening and took away Linda's body. He explained the process and some of the decisions that had to be made. An appointment was arranged for me to attend the funeral parlour the next morning.

It was sad to see the space in the bed, where Linda had fought the cancer to her last breath. Emotionally, I think I was on autopilot for most of the time. From time to time, the reality hit me and I would let the tears flow for a moment, before returning to whatever task lay ahead. Everyone left, leaving just Iain and me in the house. Eventually Iain retired to his bed with the agreement that I could call on him if I needed him. I settled down for the night, with an empty single bed beside me. I felt God's presence in the space that Linda had occupied and was comforted by the assurance that **He** would never leave me. I slept fitfully and rose early on the Friday to face another day.

I had my meeting with the funeral director and his assistant, a lovely lady called Alison. It was difficult because tears were never far from me. Linda's funeral was set for six days time on Thursday October 29th at 9.45am. Linda had said that she wanted to be cremated and I knew that when my time came, I personally wanted to be buried. We had not really discussed this mismatch, because we did not think her death was imminent. The main reason that Linda gave for wanting to be cremated was that she did not want people to stand in the cold beside a graveside. I judged that she did not have particularly strong feelings, so I took the "executive decision" and opted for a burial.

Later that day Stuart arrived from the USA and I collected him at Glasgow Airport. I was glad to have my eldest son back home. Fraser was to arrive on the Saturday and my brother Dave and his wife Alison were flying in on the Monday.

Over the weekend our house was really busy, with visits from so many people wanting to offer their condolences. Malcolm, Margaret, Linda's mum, neighbours, work colleagues, other family members and friends all visited. These were really precious times for me. It was strange, because they came to minister to me in my pain and loss, but invariably it would turn into a two way process, with us ministering to each other.

As the weekend progressed, I was open to God's leading as far as the funeral arrangements were concerned. My father had died four years previously and I had let others conduct the funeral. I had marvelled at how some people, in the midst of their grief, were able to hold things together enough to partic-ipate in the service. I remember thinking, *I could never, ever do that.* I knew that I would have been overcome with my emotions and it would have been very uncomfortable for the mourners. So I had left it to others to conduct his funeral. I knew what my dad wanted and had been involved in arranging the format of the service, but had stopped short of participating. My cousin John had conducted my dad's funeral and another cousin Billy delivered the eulogy. The service went really well and was a fine tribute to him.

I began to realise that for Linda's funeral I wanted to be more involved. I had a strong sense of what I believed Linda would have wanted and also what I wanted. Steve was to lead the service and I met with him. I had been present at a number of Christian funerals, where I had cringed at the language used in reference to non believers. I wanted Linda's funeral to be an inclusive affair, where anyone, no matter what their belief, could come and mourn. Many of the "angels" who had helped us on our journey were not Christians and had enriched our lives, serving us with open hearts. Steve smiled graciously and said that he would bear it in mind. The meeting went well and a broad structure was agreed.

The funeral was to include Ian, the rector from the Episcopal Church in Hamilton. I had grown very close to many of the people there (especially through Linda's illness) and wanted them to be officially represented. He was a very gracious man and had visited me on a number of occasions during Linda's illness. I had found solace for my soul in some of his wise comments. However as I considered what I wanted, I realised that my preference for a representative was not for Ian, but for one of the other priests, a wonderful man called John McLeod. Through the years we had developed a special bond and I seemed to sense God's leading; that John was to be the one. I met with Ian and explained what I wanted and he readily agreed. Another person could have taken offence, but I had the confidence in Ian, to know that he would accept this gracefully.

During this time I also had a surprising leading, as regards who might take Linda's eulogy.

It could be me!

I did a bit of wrestling with God in regards to this, but in the end I opened myself at least to the possibility. I started to address how I was going to achieve it. My thoughts turned to my voice coach, Deidre. She had guided me through a number of musical adventures, which had turned out to be very meaningful experiences. She knew me well and how emotional I could get. I felt that if she thought that I could do it and was willing to coach me through the process, then I had a chance of pulling it off.

I had never been a confident public speaker or reader and Deirdre and I had done some work to change that, so that

I now found that it was possible for me to enjoy reading in public. At that time I remembered Linda voicing her puzzlement, as to the reason for my working in this particular area. I had replied that for some reason I just *"knew"* that I had to do it. Now it began to make sense.

Time was short, as Deirdre had been on holiday and had just come back on Saturday. I telephoned her and we discussed what I was considering. After giving it some thought she gave her opinion.

"I think you could do it, but it is a big ask of yourself. Compose something and we can get together on Monday at noon."

On Saturday evening, I set about preparing what I would like to say and found it difficult to compose something that was worthy of Linda. I sensed that somehow this eulogy was to be different, but I did not know how. This was a familiar feeling and I drew on my experience of preparing essays for various courses, which I had completed in the last few years. When I hit a block, I would sit by my computer and prepare notes for a "normal" essay. Then I would have to "sit on it" to get the inspiration of how to deliver it. When the inspiration came, the composition would normally flow. I had noticed that often the inspiration would come in the middle of the night. Trusting this process, I gathered up my notes, committed it into God's hands and retired to bed.

I woke in the wee hours of the morning and returned to the fray. When I thought about the eulogy I realised that my focus had been all about what **I** could remember of Linda's life. What had I learned recently about when things were about "me"? *"Take my eyes off myself and on to others"*. Then the inspiration came! The tribute to Linda was to come from everyone, including me. They would all come to the funeral with their own memories of her. My eulogy was to facilitate each one of them to recall their own memories.

My creative juices were flowing now. When those gathered came with their memories, what then? I drew on my experience of our journey together. At the end of each night we would review the happenings of the day; remember; then we would lift up our hearts and give thanks.

This would to be the structure of my eulogy. I would start it by admitting the limitations in my remembering. Different groups of people would then be addressed and I would encourage them to do their own remembering using the pattern,

Remember - lift up your hearts - and give thanks.

I would then finish with some personal reflections, including the time when I sang Linda a love song.

Everything seemed to fit perfectly, but there was one other challenge in store for me.

Perhaps I could sing her our love song as part of my eulogy? Surely not!

I was on a roll now. Perhaps I could even sing the 23rd Psalm at the graveside.

Periodically during the next day (Sunday), I would return to the eulogy and refine the content. By the time I met Deirdre on the Monday, I was satisfied that it was a beautiful piece of work. There was also an emerging awareness that part of my responsibility was to seek to create a safe space for other people to mourn.

Chapter 15
Monday and Tuesday, October 26th-27th, - Preparations for the Eulogy

On Monday at noon I attended my appointment with Deirdre. It was good to see her again and my tears flowed. She reiterated her opinion that it was indeed a "hard ask" of myself, but just maybe I could do it all; Eulogy; Love Song and the 23rd Psalm. However there was no easy way to do this and she outlined two principles that were essential to the success of the venture.

Firstly it was important that I did not enter into the emotion of the occasion. "Allow emotions to overcome you and you are a goner," she stated. Then when Deirdrie heard that my sons planned to compose and show a DVD of Linda's life, accompanied by beautiful music, at the start of the service, she was adamant. "That is for others to hear and see; listen to that and you're doomed." I was shocked by her words. "You can watch it afterwards," she quipped. Secondly the success of the venture, like all the other work that I did with Deirdre, was dependent on 'preparation, preparation and more preparation'. We did not have much time as the funeral service loomed on Thursday, just three days away.

I had the eulogy printed out in large print and Deirdre asked me to stand at the music stand and deliver it, just as I would be doing at the funeral service. I did not get very far before I was reduced to tears. She gradually coached me through the delivery of the text, concentrating on the technical aspects of it, i.e. the pace, diction, emphasis and breathing. Potentially emotional points were identified and strategies were devised to overcome them. I felt encouraged.

We then turned to the love song, Edelweiss. I thought that since I knew the song and had performed it privately to Linda and also in a church setting, that it wouldn't be quite so difficult. How wrong I was! The reading of the eulogy was easy compared to this. Again and again I was reduced to tears as memories of my beloved overwhelmed me. However Deirdre continued to patiently work with me along the same lines as the eulogy and I started to see some progress. We finished off the session by doing some work on the 23rd Psalm.

Deirdre advised me to work diligently with it and we arranged another session for the next day, Tuesday at 4.30pm. It was also important to practise the songs with the organist, a close friend called Doris. I had already anticipated this and had arranged to meet up with her later that evening in the Baptist Church.

Our friendship with Doris and her husband Jim had spanned many years and we had spent countless enjoyable evenings together. Doris was a wonderful cook and after feeding us, we would spend time relaxing and talking together until the wee small hours of the morning. We had always felt comfortable with them and would share our feelings openly with each other. During Linda's illness they had been very much a part of our support group. Doris was an accomplished pianist with a lovely touch and flow to her playing and I felt that she was the ideal person to help me negotiate this "hard ask".

The practice with Doris did not start well. Time and time again after a few lines, I would be reduced to tears. After about half an hour of this, I remember Doris stopping and asking in gentle exasperation, "Do you really have to do this?"

I sought to reassure her, "Doris I know I can do this. Just trust me."

As time went on, we began to see some progress and I arranged to see her again the next evening, after Deirdre's session. We both recognised that there was not much time, as the funeral was to take place in 2 ½ days' time.

Even although it was a really busy time for me, I was able to snatch periods to work on the draft of the eulogy. I seemed to have the assurance that it would be OK. Different insights came and I was astounded at the process. Gradually I refined the wording of the eulogy until it was just right. Thereafter it was just a case of practising the delivery.

I was also open to understand my limitations and was aware that the "big ask" could be trimmed. This proved to be the case with my plan to sing the 23rd Psalm. It came to me when I was practising it, that I did not have to do it. I realised that one of the reasons for including it was that I felt a bit guilty about overriding Linda's wish to be cremated. It was my gesture to her that even if the rain was pouring down and the mourners experiencing discomfort, it could still be a special part of the service. Once this motivation was out in the open, I was able to let it go and I felt that a burden had been lifted from my shoulders. I would arrange for someone else to lead the singing of the Psalm.

Up until this point, I had planned to deliver the eulogy, which included the singing of the love song. I soon realised that this would be too much for me and possibly even for the congregation. The eulogy text was lovely, just by itself and would take place early in the service. The congregation would need time to absorb it. The love song with its beautiful introductory story would take place at the end of the service. It would be a fitting send off for Linda. My "big ask" was now broken down into two more manageable portions and it seemed perfect!

My second appointment with Deidre was for 4.30pm on the Tuesday and it had to be the last one before the funeral. Stuart asked if he could accompany me and I willingly agreed. I was glad to have him with me and wondered what he would make of Deirdre.

After the introductions, he sat on the couch in the music room and did not say a word throughout the session. I showed Deirdre the finished text of my eulogy and she remarked, "this is a beautiful, insightful piece of work!"

We worked away at it and the process went relatively smoothly, with a few amendments from Deirdre. Emotional hotspots were identified and strategies devised to avoid or diffuse them.

Deirdre agreed with my decision to trim down my musical participation. Given the situation, it was really good to only have one "well kent" song to work on. Edelweiss's introductory story posed no insurmountable problems, but singing it and remaining in control proved very emotionally demanding. I still broke down. However, as we worked on it, the occasions reduced in frequency. Deirdre commented that while it would not be the "end of the world" if I broke down at sometime during my delivery, it would be better if I could remain in control. I would feel so much better afterwards and it would be far more effective. When the session ended, I felt a growing confidence that with God's help; I might just pull it off.

When Stuart and I travelled back in the car, he voiced his astonishment at the session. He had sat there mesmerised, watching our process in action. Nothing was "rocket science". It was just so simple and effective and he found Deirdre to be an amazing teacher. He was used to teaching students at the university where he worked, but this was something different.

After dinner I met with Doris for the final practice of Edelweiss. I faltered a bit during the first couple of attempts, but at least I did not break down. Using Deirdre's techniques, I worked on my delivery and by the end of the session, I was able to sing it effectively and in control of my emotions. My confidence increased, but I realised that it all teetered on a knife edge. I could now sing it right through without breaking down in an empty church, but how would I be with a bulging congregation?

Chapter 16
Further preparations for the Funeral

The arrangements for the funeral service were taking shape and I left a lot of the practicalities to my three sons. They were all staying with me and I was glad to leave the composition for the funeral leaflet to them. All being very computer literate they composed a lovely proof. I wanted it to be printed professionally and so they arranged for a local printer to produce the final product. The Northumbrian Offices Liturgy had been a tremendous spiritual resource to us both, throughout Linda's illness. I came up with the idea of getting individual sections of it enlarged and laminated by the printer. The plan was to have these displayed on the walls of the back hall in the church, where the funeral meal would be served. Linda's memorial DVD was almost ready. It consisted of photographs of Linda's life, set to beautiful music.

An estimate was needed on the numbers that would attend the funeral. I briefly considered transferring it to the much larger Episcopal Church, but rejected the notion. The really close ties were with the Baptist folks and so it just had to be held there. The church could hold up to 150 and we were estimating that there may be double that number coming. It was becoming evident that it would be a tight squeeze in the wee Baptist sanctuary.

The school where Linda had worked organised a bus to transfer staff to the church, even though they were situated just a mile away. The demand was so great that they had to cancel lessons and arrange for replacement staff. Linda had touched so many lives in our community, that we were overwhelmed by the response. It appeared that everybody wanted to attend and we were constantly giving the advice to "arrive early if you want a seat".

During this time, I had a visit from my cousin John and his lovely wife Catherine. They had been a tremendous support to me after the death of my father. Dad had requested that John lead his funeral service and I remembered John visiting me to make the arrangements. He had asked whether I wanted my dad's coffin to be inside the church, or left outside in the hearse, as was the growing practice. I had not even considered leaving it outside and John commented that it seemed strange to him. "What was the point of having a funeral service with everybody there except the person who had died?"

I had concurred and my dad had "attended" his own funeral. During John's visit, the subject came up and I told him that Linda would also be "attending" her own funeral.

Around this time arrangements had been made for Linda's body to be viewed at the undertakers and my eldest son, Stuart, indicated that he also wanted to be there. I attended with some trepidation, but also with a sense of anticipation at seeing my beloved for one last time. To my surprise, I was shocked by her appearance. The body I was viewing did not look like my Linda at all! I felt distraught, but was able to hide my feelings from Alison, the undertaker's assistant. They had probably spent a great deal of time and effort in the preparation of the body and she seemed so pleased at the finished product. I didn't have the heart to tell her how I really felt, so I thanked her for her service and left.

Once outside I was able to share my feelings with Stuart. One thing was glaringly obvious to me. That was not Linda! It was her body, but her spirit wasn't in it! I felt distraught, *Where was she then?* I returned home and shared how I felt about the body with the others. I became involved in the busyness of the household, but all the time inwardly I was asking myself the question. It seemed important for me to come to some understanding about this.

I phoned Steve and he came round later in the afternoon. He listened attentively to my dilemma. "If Linda wasn't in her body, was she in the room unseen? Could she hear what we were saying? Was it possible to feel her presence? Was she in heaven looking down, or was she in some other place, out of contact with us all?" I knew that these probably were unanswerable questions, but I was struggling and seemed to need a workable understanding.

I expected that Steve would turn to the Bible for answers, but instead he turned to a point of view from Jewish tradition and offered it to me.

"The Jews have a period of structured mourning which lasts for seven days. During the first three days some believe that the deceased soul is still present and visitors are not supposed to offer any words of comfort or sorrow. They are there to share grief rather than try to analyse it. They can weep and mourn with you, but should not speak unless directly addressed or asked to. After the third day it is believed that the person's soul has departed and they can begin to speak more freely. The custom is about shared grief and respecting the right to grieve and to wail if needed."

He knew me well enough to sense that quoting the familiar Bible verses to me would probably not be helpful and he was right. Somehow his words soothed my troubled soul. I thanked God for sending this "big bearded angel" into my life.

My continuing concern was to make the church as safe a place as possible for people to come and mourn for Linda. Space was at a premium and there would have to be adequate room at the front for the coffin. With my experience of viewing Linda's body fresh in my mind, it suddenly occurred to me that the place for Linda's coffin was outside the church. It was Linda's lovely body that was in the coffin, not her spirit. I respected her body and would treat it with due reverence, but it was an empty shell. Her spirit would be inside the church and in all our hearts. It just seemed so right and I knew that she would understand and approve. This would have the added advantage of freeing up a lot of space at the front of the church and avoid the situation of mourners being squeezed into the close proximity of the coffin.

As the funeral itself loomed nearer, I seemed to be able to trust in God that it would be alright. The house was very busy with a steady stream of people offering their condolences. A pattern started to emerge. They would arrive, very often not knowing what to say or how to minister to me and I would usually end up ministering to them in some way. In this environment of shared vulnerability, invariably a *"meeting"* of souls would take place, with us ministering to each other. This would be a precious time and we would part with full hearts.

During this time I seemed to get an inner strength and clarity of thought. I was still in a very vulnerable state and from time to time would be overwhelmed by emotion. My strategy was just to let the tears come and then move on. The main focus for me was on the funeral service and celebrating Linda's life. Perhaps by God's grace we could make it a meaningful experience for all.

Chapter 17
The Funeral Service

The day of the service came. Much preparation had gone into the funeral by so many people. My sons had finished the beautiful order of service and memorial DVD. David had generously donated a wonderful display of flowers and the Baptist Church folk had all worked tirelessly to prepare the church for the service and meal afterwards.

Steve and I had gone over the order of service and so I informed participants of their duties. I recognised that this would be a difficult service for Steve to take, since he had such a close relationship with Linda, but I was confident that he would be able to hold it together. After having one last practice in my bedroom at home, I committed the whole undertaking into God's hands.

Lachlan had travelled up early from Dumfries. He had arranged a viewing of Linda's body at the funeral parlour and wanted to see her for one last time. The family group consisted of Stuart, Fraser and Iain; Dave and Alison; Gran, Malcolm and Margaret and Lachlan. Roger, who had accompanied me on the piano and was my daughter in law's father, also indicated that he wanted to be part of the family group. Although he was not a direct family member, I was pleased to have him sit with us.

We arrived at the church and were astounded by the turn out. It was 10 minutes before the service was due to start and the church was already bulging at the seams. It was lovely to see so many well loved faces wherever I looked. As we filed in, I looked out for Roger and beckoned him to join me. He looked relieved and sat beside me. People continued to stream in and fill every available space. I reflected upon my decision to leave Linda's coffin outside and thanked God for His leading. The vestibule at the entrance of the church was also full with some mourners spilling out into the car park.

I focused on my task in hand. My main function was to deliver the eulogy and sing the love song. It was really important for me to remain calm and not enter into the emotion of the situation.

The service started with a welcome and introduction from Steve. He said that it was understandable that, "We have come here in our shared grief and pain and common sense of loss. However, it is the family's wish that this is to be a celebration of Linda's life and beauty, physical and spiritual. God had not allowed her to have a long, lingering death, but had taken her quickly. From Linda's point of view, this had been one last breath here and her first breath in eternity. Closing her eyes in sleep here and awakening in the presence of her Lord".

We then sang Linda's favourite hymn, which we had sung at our wedding. It was "How great Thou art" and was lovely. The last words perhaps reflected Linda's experience,

"And take me home - what joy shall fill my heart!

Then I shall bow in humble adoration

and there proclaim my God, how great Thou art."

John McLeod read from Genesis chapter 2, which spoke of the beauty of creation. It was wonderful to hear his rich voice delivering it. He then led in prayer. Afterwards David told me that he had been transfixed by John's face towards the end of his prayer. "It seemed to be lit up like an angel's". That's why John had to be there instead of the rector, Ian – it was for David's sake!

Linda's memorial video was then played. I longed to see it, but alas, I could not watch it. I sat in my seat, covered my ears and avoided looking at any of the wonderful photographs that were being flashed up on the screen. I had a task in hand and it was important to stay focussed so I consoled myself with the promise to view the DVD at home later. A collective appreciative sigh was uttered by the congregation at the end of the presentation.

Steve then talked about the close relationship he had with Linda. He had always wanted a sister and ended up with three younger brothers. In his dealings with her, he had come to know her *as the sister he had always wanted*. He then read the beautiful passage from Proverbs chapter 31, which began with *"Who can find a virtuous woman? For her price is far above rubies"*. As he described this "virtuous woman", it fitted Linda like a glove, capturing her essence.

It was time for me to deliver the eulogy. When Steve introduced me, I took a deep breath and made my way to the podium at the front of the church. I organised my notes and looked up to address the congregation.

The church was packed solid with mourners and it was stiflingly hot. My heart went out to all our friends gathered in this atmosphere. I paused, commented on this, took off my jacket and invited any who felt inclined to do the same. I sensed an easing of the tension in myself and in the congregation.

Chapter 18
Eulogy for Linda Margaret Loch

(Transcript of the eulogy I delivered, bold type words emphasised)

That was a **lovely** commemorative video. I am sure we all agree; Linda was a **beautiful** person in every way.

She was 58 when she passed on and we have all been **privileged to** know her at **different** stages of her **sweet** life and in **different capacities**. I volunteered to do this eulogy, but I only knew her for **41** years. Perhaps between us, as we reflect together in our **hearts**, we can cover the whole **58 years**.

I am aware that this could be an emotional experience for us all, so I am going to suggest a **simple** way to help us all experience it **fully**, without becoming overcome with emotion. Linda and I used to do this at the end of each night. We would remember all the **wonderful** things we had seen and experienced **that** day. Then we would lift up our **hearts** and give **thanks**.

Linda's mum Margaret, Billy and Cathy – you knew her for the whole 58 years as a daughter, and niece. We didn't know her as a baby. What was she like? Maybe you can tell us about it afterwards. She sure looked a **sweet** thing.

Remember, lift up your hearts and give thanks.

Malcolm she was your sister, for 56 years. What was she like? Linda was a **very tidy** person and I remember her telling me, that once she got **so** angry with you that she **attacked** you with the **hoover**. When her **dander** was up, she was a formidable person.

Remember, lift up your heart and give thanks.

Mary, you knew her when she started her first job in the insurance office in Edinburgh. What was she like? Just out of school, perhaps full of fear, insecurities and *excitement*. You have remained close friends for the past *42 years*. What was it *about her* that made it a *pleasure* for us to meet three or four times a year for a meal? The time seemed to pass so quickly didn't it?

Remember, lift up your heart and give thanks.

Stuart, Fraser and Iain, she was your mother. I was your father, making my way in life, very busy with a career and church responsibilities. You are the young people that you are today, *mainly* because of her *influence*. What was she like? I *don't think* you could have asked for a *better mum*.

Remember, lift up your hearts and give thanks.

David, my brother, Alison my sister in law and Margaret my other sister in law. You have all known her for a *long* time. What were your *first* impressions? What was she like?

Remember, lift up your hearts and give thanks.

This is a wonderful wee church, full to the brim with *love* and *compassion*. Janet, Helen, Vida, Edith, Joan and Andrew to name a few. Trevor and Freda, the pastor and his wife when we first came, Jim Gordon and Shiela. All of the folks that have come since, knowing Linda for varying lengths of time, *especially* Steve, Chris, sweet Rebecca and Philip. What was it about Linda that makes you *smile* when you hear her name *now*?

Remember, lift up your hearts and give thanks.

Jim and Doris and Lachlan, neighbours in Greenhall Place and beyond. She *touched* you didn't she?

Remember, lift up your hearts and give thanks.

Friends and Colleagues at the school, where Linda worked for the past 13 years, especially Jeanette, Myra, Janice and all the rest of the girls in the office. Teachers and other staff. Why was it that this was **one** funeral you didn't want to miss?

Remember, lift up your hearts and give thanks.

Everyone can relax now. I won't be mentioning anyone else's name.

I am **sorry** for putting you all on the spot, but I would not subject you to something that I would not subject **myself** to.

What was **my** experience of Linda over the 41 years that I knew her?

She was **just** a **beautiful person**, but I didn't **always** recognise that.

About 15 years ago, she put me on the spot and asked me. "Do you think I am **beautiful**"?

I tried to answer this honestly, because Linda had an **uncanny knowledge** of knowing when I was not being fully truthful, as I saw it. I probably understood beauty at the time as someone who was stunningly attractive physically and I replied, I thought that she was **lovely**, but perhaps not **beautiful**. I remember seeing a **fleeting sadness** in her eyes and then it was gone. She was **so** courageous to ask that question. You see, she just wanted to be told **honestly** that she was **beautiful**, but unfortunately she asked the **wrong** person at the **wrong** time.

I am sorry to say that it took the diagnosis of breast cancer for me to at last recognise the **full beauty** of Linda. I took my eyes off myself and was able to see her as she really was – a **beautiful human being**. You know the concept of having a swear box, put 10p in the box every time you swear. Well I am pleased to say that during the last 9 months of her life here with us, if I had put a 10p in the box every time I told her I loved her, or that she was so beautiful, **I would be bankrupt** by now. She died at peace and I believe, in no doubt of her beauty.

It is a **lovely** story, but it is also sad. Why did it have to take the diagnosis of **cancer** for that to happen?

Perhaps each one of us wants to be told that we are **beautiful**, but this desire is hidden so far below, we don't recognise it.

Can I share a **secret** that both Linda and I found when we were journeying together through this **difficult** time?

We found that if we took our minds off **ourselves** and really looked for the **beauty** in **others**, lo and behold it was there to be seen. At the end of the day, when we were doing our quiet time before God, we would say, *"what a lovely person so and so was"* and we would give thanks. Instead of complaining about people, or our lot in life, once our eyes were taken off **ourselves and** on to **others**, we were able **see** their beauty. And you know, when we did that, they returned the favour and saw our beauty and we were all enriched. No wonder our prevailing emotion was one of thankfulness, despite what was happening medically. We found ourselves **rich** beyond **measure**.

Perhaps even **now**, we can reflect on our families and friends and **even** those sitting next to us in the pews. Can we take our eyes off ourselves long enough to want to connect with them and see their beauty? It's a risky business, but perhaps it's worth a try. You might just become aware of your **own** beauty within you.

Chapter 19
Funeral Service - Ending

I felt that my delivery of the eulogy had gone extremely well and seemed to be appreciated by the congregation. As I returned to my seat I thanked God for Deirdre, as I could not have done it without her assistance. I also thanked God for His help in leading me a step at a time, giving me the inspiration to write it and the courage to deliver it. However I realised that my task was still only half done and it was important not to lose my focus.

Steve then led prayers of intercession. His sermon was based on a passage from 1st Peter Chapter 3. He summed up his thoughts on this passage," As we think of Linda, we celebrate, remember and give thanks for the unfading beauty of a gentle and quiet spirit, which is of real worth in God's sight. One last breath here… and the next in eternity".

Steve then read from 1 Corinthians 15:35-44. He commented that "the family need to know that what you saw at the end is not what she is now in Christ. The body that is sown perishable is raised imperishable; the body that is sown in dishonour is raised in honour; the body that is sown in frail flesh is raised immortal. That beautiful person, Linda, who we were privileged to know for a while here, now blossoms in God's presence: a precious flower opening up in the very sight of God with her true beauty revealed".

Echoes of my desperate questioning, *Where is Linda now?* and my previous meeting with Steve came to the fore. There was certainly one member of the family that *"needed to know"*. I felt encouraged.

The final part of my blessed task lay ahead: Singing the love song, Edelweiss. Once again I steeled myself to what lay ahead and made my way to the lectern. I felt remarkably calm and composed. There were two parts to this; a beautiful introductory story and the actual song itself. I smiled at Doris, who was ready at the piano and began.

Introduction to Edelweiss

(The transcript of my introduction, bold type words are emphasised)

Linda used to complain to me that I **never** gave her presents.

She was **right** and I always felt guilty when she said that and resolved to start buying her **impromptu** presents. However I very rarely did and the **main** reason **was** that I **never** knew what to buy her.

Now I have my dad's **genes** in me and he was the one who gave my mum a **torch** for her **Birthday**. Needless to say, she was **not best pleased**, but perhaps that gives you an **insight** into my struggle.

However during the last few weeks of Linda's life, I **found** a present that **no one else** could give her and she **loved** it.

I started to sing her **Love** songs in the morning.

The first one I tried was one I loved and it reminded me **so** much of **her**.

I started with **Edelweiss**.

At first, I could only get a **couple** of words out, before both of us descended into **floods** of tears. The only way I could **do** it was if I looked out of the window and she looked down at the floor. However with perseverance and with the training that I had from my voice coach, Deirdre, I was **eventually** able to sing it **right through**, looking into her **eyes.** It was a **wonderful** experience and I went on to sing her **other** love songs.

Now near the end of the service, I would like to sing it to her **one more time** and I would like **you** to help me.

If I may, I would like to suggest a way of **visualising** this, to help us control our emotions.

Linda is **not** in the coffin. That is why her coffin is **not here**. Her spirit is with **God**. Perhaps if we visualise **Linda** looking down on us **all** and if we take our eyes off **ourselves**, look up and **follow** the words as they rise up to her, we **might just** do it. It would be **lovely** for **us** to give **her** that **last beautiful present**.

I intend to sing it through once and then perhaps, **you** could help me by **humming** it, as I sing it again.

Deirdre had taught me well; I managed to deliver the introduction and sing the beautiful song all the way through, remaining composed throughout. As I sang the words of the song, they seemed to rise up to heaven. I invited people to *"hum",* as I sang it through a second time. Some did, but many also softly sung it and a beautiful communal offering rose up in tribute to Linda and in thanksgiving to God. It was a wonderful experience and I thanked God for this moment of Grace.

The "hard ask" had been accomplished and I felt the glow of satisfaction of having done a good job well. Hopefully I had contributed to bringing a lovely tribute to my beloved and had helped to make this space a safe place for all our friends and family to come and grieve.

Steve encouraged us by quoting Paul's letter to the Philippians, where he reminded them that "their citizenship was in heaven". He commented, "As Linda awakes to the new dawn in her homeland we rejoice with her and give thanks. God our Father now holds her in the palm of His hands and surrounds her with His love".

We finished this part of the service by singing another one of Linda's favourite hymns, which had the opening lines;

"How deep the Father's love for us

How vast beyond all measure".

These words summed up Linda's attitude to her Creator and the relationship she had with Him.

Steve pronounced the benediction from the Book of Numbers.

"The LORD bless you and keep you; the LORD make His face to shine upon you and be gracious to you: the LORD turn His face towards you and give you peace".

The service had finished and the congregation remained standing to allow the family group to pass down the aisle. I stood up and caught Doris's eye as she played the closing refrains. We had done it together and I raised my fist in salute to her. As ever, she had played beautifully during the service and I was so grateful to have her as a friend. I felt a great sense of relief, that my active participation in the service was over and I could leave the remainder of it in the hands of my dear friends.

The family group squeezed their way down one of the aisles, through the vestibule and out into the car park. There must have been about 100 people in the car park. It was only then I realised that most of them had not been able to get into the church. There was so many "well-kent" faces everywhere I looked. We had decided beforehand that it was not practical to follow the custom of the funeral party shaking hands with all the mourners at the end of the service. However I was so grateful to all these lovely people that I started shaking their hands anyway. I was aware of the funeral party waiting for me, but I just took time to give each my thanks.

Eventually I managed to tear myself away and joined the others in the main funeral car. I had just taken my seat when out of the corner of my eye I spotted two dear friends of mine that I had missed. Sarah and Helen were part of a counselling professional development group that I had attended four weekends a year for the past five years. We had grown very close during this time and both had encouraged me greatly. I had not been able to meet with them since Linda's diagnosis and it was so great to see them.

On the spur of the moment I stopped the car, tore out and gave them both a hug. There was something about Sarah in particular, that required this response. Previously I had found out that we were distantly related (her mother was also a Loch) and I had the sense of a "sisterly"relationship with her (not unlike Steve's relationship with Linda, as "the sister he never had").

Chapter 20
Funeral service – Graveside

We respectfully gathered round the graveside. I kept on seeing people that I did not expect to be there and felt so happy for their presence. Thankfully the weather had remained dry. It was good to have the open space for all the people to gather.

The service was brief and in many ways a condensed version of the church service, except without my involvement.

Steve spoke of the "comfort of Scripture" and "the joy that is now Linda's, taking one last breath here and her first breath in eternity".

There was a scripture reading from Revelation 7:14-17, which promised that God would *"wipe away every tear from our eyes"*.

After a simple prayer of thanksgiving for Linda's life and ministry, there was another Scripture reading from Romans 8:35-39. It contained the assurance that nothing would be able to *"separate us from the love of God, which is in Christ Jesus our Lord"*.

Steve encouraged us to have the right perspective and that for Linda, "this is an end to suffering and the beginning of glory; the simple exchange of one last breath here, for her first breath in eternity".

It was time to lay Linda's body to rest. The undertaker shouted out the names of those who would lower her into the ground. Each stepped forward in turn to take hold of their cords. Apart from me, there was my brother Dave, my sons, Stuart, Fraser and Iain, Linda's brother Malcolm, Linda's uncle Billy and Lachlan. It was lovely to have all these wonderful people around me, as we lowered her body into the ground.

Steve gave the committal, which included the familiar words,

"For as much as it has pleased Almighty God, of his great mercy, to receive unto himself the soul of our dear sister Linda here departed, we therefore commit her body to the ground, earth to earth, ashes to ashes, dust to dust; in the sure and certain hope of the resurrection to eternal life, through our Lord Jesus Christ."

We then sang the 23rd Psalm to the haunting melody of the Scottish tune, Crimond. The singing was led by another two of our dearest friends, Rev John MacSporran and Jim Simpson. I had intended to sing this as a solo and I was so thankful to hear their wonderful voices give us all the starting notes.

The words were so beautiful and summed up so much of our Journey together and God's provision for us. As we sang it the words of the psalm rose up to heaven.

The Lord's my shepherd, I'll not want;
He makes me down to lie
In pastures green; He leadeth me
The quiet waters by.
My soul He doth restore again,
And me to walk doth make
Within the paths of righteousness,
E'en for His own name sake.
Yea though I walk in death's dark vale
Yet will I fear no ill:
For Thou art with me, and Thy rod
And staff me comfort still.
My table Thou hast furnished
In presence of my foes;
My head thou dost with oil anoint
And my cup overflows.

Goodness and mercy all my life
Shall surely follow me;
And in God's house for evermore
My dwelling place shall be.

Scottish Psalter 1650

Steve pronounced the Benediction from 2 Corinthians 13:14 *"The grace of the Lord Jesus Christ, the love of God and the fellowship of the Holy Spirit be with you now and evermore, Amen".*

The tradition in Scotland is that the undertaker invites mourners to throw some soil from a container down on to the coffin as a last farewell. Linda just loved pink carnations and I added to that tradition by arranging a supply of carnations to be available. As my soil clattered on her casket, followed by her favourite flower, I said my final goodbye to my love and my heart was filled with sadness. Others followed my lead and it was a beautiful way to end the service.

Our Journey was now complete. What a terrible and beautiful Journey it turned out to be!

Did God keep His promise, that He had given us eight months previously?

"I say this because I know what I am planning for you", says the Lord. "I have good plans for you not to hurt you. I will give you hope and a good future"

Jeremiah 29:11

I leave you to decide!

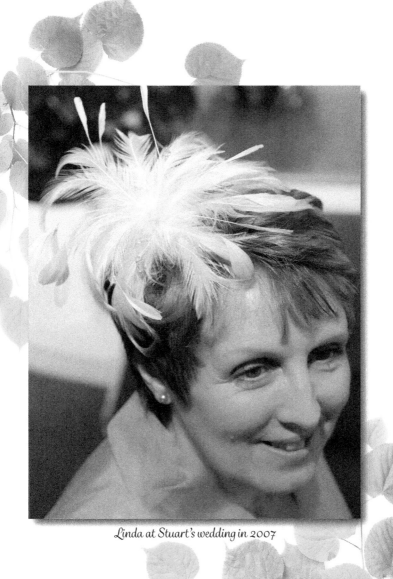

Linda at Stuart's wedding in 2007

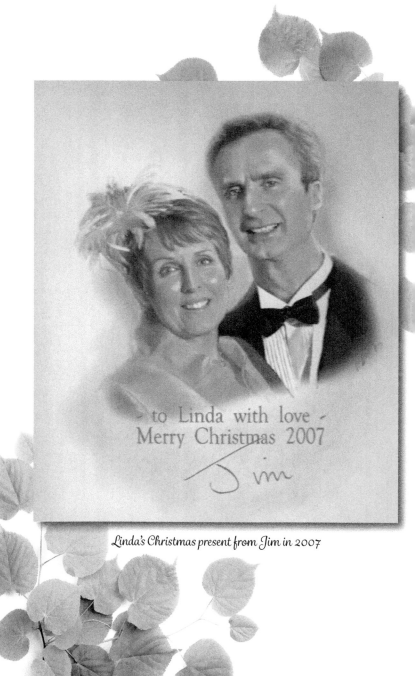

- to Linda with love -
Merry Christmas 2007

Jim

Linda's Christmas present from Jim in 2007

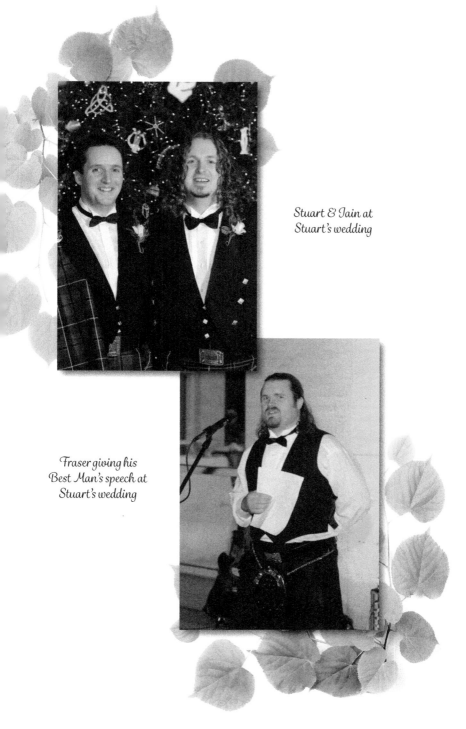

Stuart & Iain at
Stuart's wedding

Fraser giving his
Best Man's speech at
Stuart's wedding

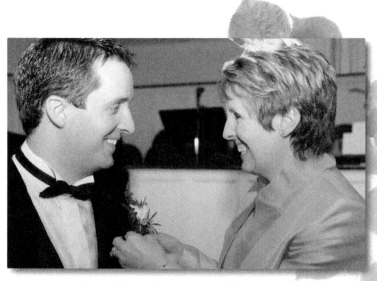

Linda helping Stuart to get ready for his big day

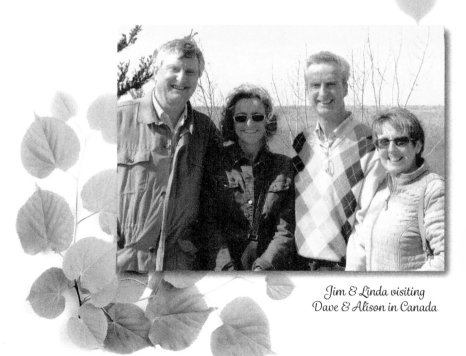

Jim & Linda visiting
Dave & Alison in Canada

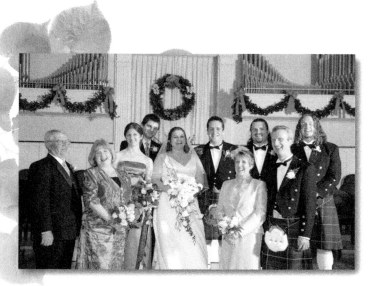

Jim, Linda & three sons with Jessica's family at Stuart's wedding

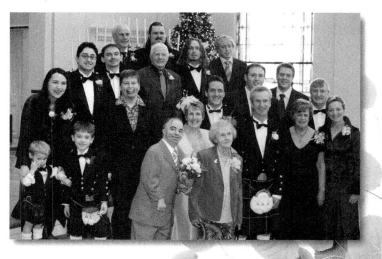

Scottish & Canadian guests at the wedding

Epilogue

*A*s I write this, it has been six and a half years since my beloved Linda was taken from me. Fraser, Larinda and their 3 children, Nathanael, Ethan and Hannah returned home from Canada the following summer and now live in in Denny-loanhead, 25 miles from me. Stuart and family have moved to Montgomery Alabama and now include an energetic wee boy called Sam. My nomadic youngest son Iain, eventually found his vocation as a teacher and the love of his life in Kim, a Southern Belle from Birmingham, Alabama. After teaching in Brazil for three years, they came back to Edinburgh in July 2014 to be married, before jetting off to Japan for a two year contract. Switzerland now beckons them.

As regards myself, it probably took me about four years to work through my grieving process. I wondered after the intensity of my spiritual journey of "Autumn Leaves", whether I would return to normal living. While this was the case in part, I am pleased to say that God continued to walk with me, through many other adventures (some of them musical), teaching me numerous lessons along the way. Wonderfully I was able to let Linda go, which enabled me to gradually build a new life for myself. This new life was based on compassion and a simple faith, where I sought to serve God by helping others, which included my family, church, The Haven, Linda's school and the local community.

A central person in my new life was Linda's mum, as Linda had been her carer and that privilege was passed on to me. How I thanked God for changing my heart toward "Great Gran"!

Our relationship blossomed and we had lots of wee escapades together. Most of them were straightforward and joyous, but a few were in very dark places, where we successfully negotiated them together. Eventually her health deteriorated and she slipped away peacefully four years later, with Malcolm, Margaret and myself holding her frail hands at her bedside.

In February 2015, I had a routine inguinal hernia operation, which went disastrously wrong and I almost died. During this time, when I was delirious with pain, I had an interesting conversation with God and another being! An emergency operation was required, where 5cm had to be cut off my damaged lower intestines. This left me really weak and I lost a stone in weight, which given my slim build, I could ill afford. Although I gradually regained my strength and weight, the whole experience shattered my confidence in the faithfulness of God's provision. Thankfully He has remained faithful to me and has brought me through this dark valley to a place where I can commit my life to Him in confidence again.

I am now 67 and as I contemplate my future, I do so with excitement, anticipation and if I am honest, a degree of apprehension. As I write this, I feel that I have got my life back again and look forward to discovering God's plan for the second part of my journey.

So many beautiful things seem to keep on happening to me and I record them on my computer. In due course I plan to publish them, should I feel God's leading.

However, I recognise that I am a vulnerable person and am thankful for another 2 verses that I feel God has given me to ponder, to help me on my way.

"God has not given me a spirit of fear, but of Power and of Love and of a sound Mind" **2 Timothy 1:7 (personalised)**.

"My Grace is sufficient for thee; for My strength is made perfect in weakness" **2 Corinthians 12:9 KJV**

P.S. For your interest, I have started dating again!

About The Author

*J*im was born in West Lothian in 1949 in the hospital where both his parents workd. He and his elder brother Dave grew up in the small, nearby village of Dechmont.. He was always drawn to the sciences and on leaving school, started his career as a Junior Medical Laboratory Technician in the hospital of his birth. After qualification, he married Linda and 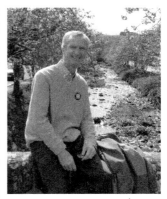 moved through to a Senior position in the Victoria Infirmary Glasgow, where he remained for the rest of his career.

He was promoted to Chief Medical Laboratory Technician at the young age of 25. Unfortunately, near the end of his career he encountered problems with depression and anxiety and was given Ill Health Retirement in 1997. He then retrained, receiving a Diploma in Counselling from Jordanhill College and gained 5 years voluntary counselling experience in the Tom Allan Centre in the centre of Glasgow. He left to take up a part time counselling position in GP practices in Lanarkshire for 2 years, before leaving to be the carer for his ailing father in the final stages of his life.

Jim and Linda had 3 sons, who at the time of this story, had all left home and were scattered throughout the world. (USA, Canada and Australia). The 2 older sons were married and had produced 5 grandchildren.

Jim has always been interested in psychological processes and has struggled through the years with his vulnerability. He has a refreshing honesty and courage and has always showed psychological insight and compassion in his dealings with people.

Lightning Source UK Ltd.
Milton Keynes UK
UKOW07f1554260816

281578UK00014B/94/P